GOLO DIET
COOKBOOK

Henry Irving

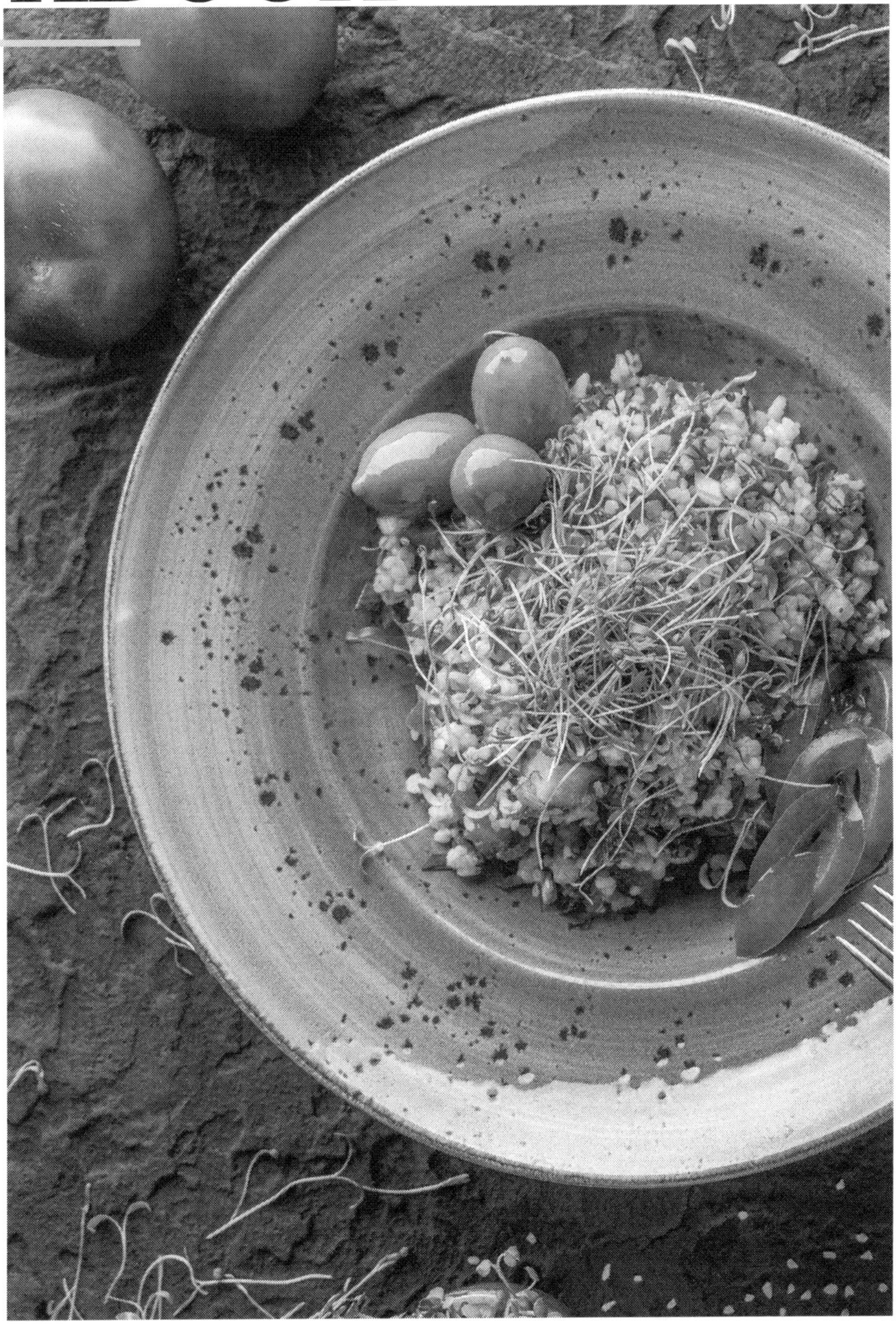

LEGAL & DISCLAIMER

The information contained in this book and its contents is not designed to replace or take the place of any form of medical or professional advice; and is not meant to replace the need for independent medical, financial, legal, or other professional advice or services, as may be required. The content and information in this book has been provided for educational and entertainment purposes only.

The content and information contained in this book has been compiled from sources deemed reliable, and it is accurate to the best of the Author's knowledge, information, and belief. However, the Author cannot guarantee its accuracy and validity and cannot be held liable for any errors and/or omissions. Further, changes are periodically made to this book as and when needed. Where appropriate and/or necessary, you must consult a professional (including but not limited to your doctor, attorney, financial advisor, or such other professional advisor) before using any of the suggested remedies, techniques, or information in this book.

Upon using the contents and information contained in this book, you agree to hold harmless the Author from and against any damages, costs, and expenses, including any legal fees potentially resulting from the application of any of the information provided by this book. This disclaimer applies to any loss, damages or injury caused by the use and application, whether directly or indirectly, of any advice or information presented, whether for breach of contract, tort, negligence, personal injury, criminal intent, or under any other cause of action. You agree to accept all risks of using the information presented inside this book.

You agree that by continuing to read this book, where appropriate and/or necessary, you shall consult a professional (including but not limited to your doctor, attorney, or financial advisor or such other advisor as needed) before using any of the suggested remedies, techniques, or information in this book.

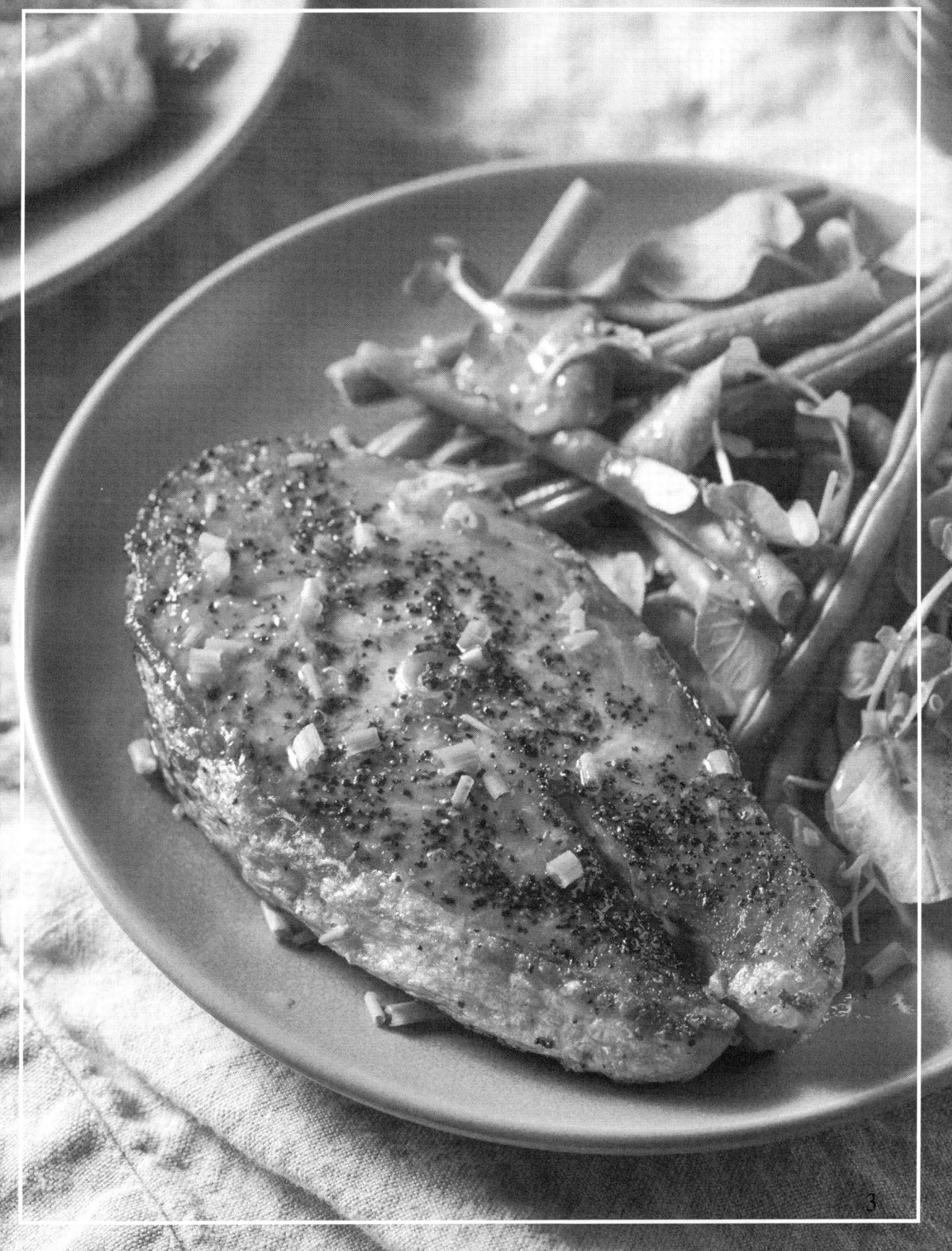

TABLE OF CONTENT

INTRODUCTION 6

WHAT IS GOLO DIET? 10

FOODS TO EAT AND AVOID 18

HEALTH BENEFITS GOLO DIET 24

GOLO DIET AND WEIGHT LOSS 28

BREAKFAST RECIPES 32

Spinach Omelet 34

Tomato And Eggs Salad 36

Veggie Breakfast Bowl 38

Cajun Tofu Scramble 40

Zucchini Pancake With Guacamole 42

Strawberry Yogurt 44

Green Eggs 46

Chia Seed Pudding 48

Edamame & Sweet Pea Hummus 50

Tomatoes And Eggs 52

Tofu Scramble Toast 54

Avocado Spread 56

Granola With Grapefruit 58

Spinach Smoothie 60

Chili Spinach Mix 62

LUNCH RECIPES 64

Vegetable Wraps 66

Mushroom Soup 68

Easy Grilled Shrimp With Avocado And Tomato 70

Radish Cucumber Salad 72

Baked Vegetables 74

Italian Tomato Soup 76

Garlic Shrimp 78

Shrimp And Strawberry Salad 80

Pasta With Broccoli 82

Quinoa With Acorn Squash & Swiss Chard 84

Chicken Couscous 86

Radish Salmon Salad 88

Shrimp Salad 90

Avocado Salmon Salad 92

Zucchini Cakes 94

Black Bean And Quinoa Salad 96

Cauliflower And Green Beans 98

Cauliflower With Sausage And Leeks Toppings 100

Tuna Salad With Avocado 102

Baked Broccoli 104

DINNER RECIPES 106

Baked Chicken With Sweet Paprika 108

Chicken Pieces 110

Sea Bass 112

Cumin Salmon 114

Shrimp Zoodles 116

Delicious Salmon 118

Cauliflower Bolognese With Zucchini Noodles 120

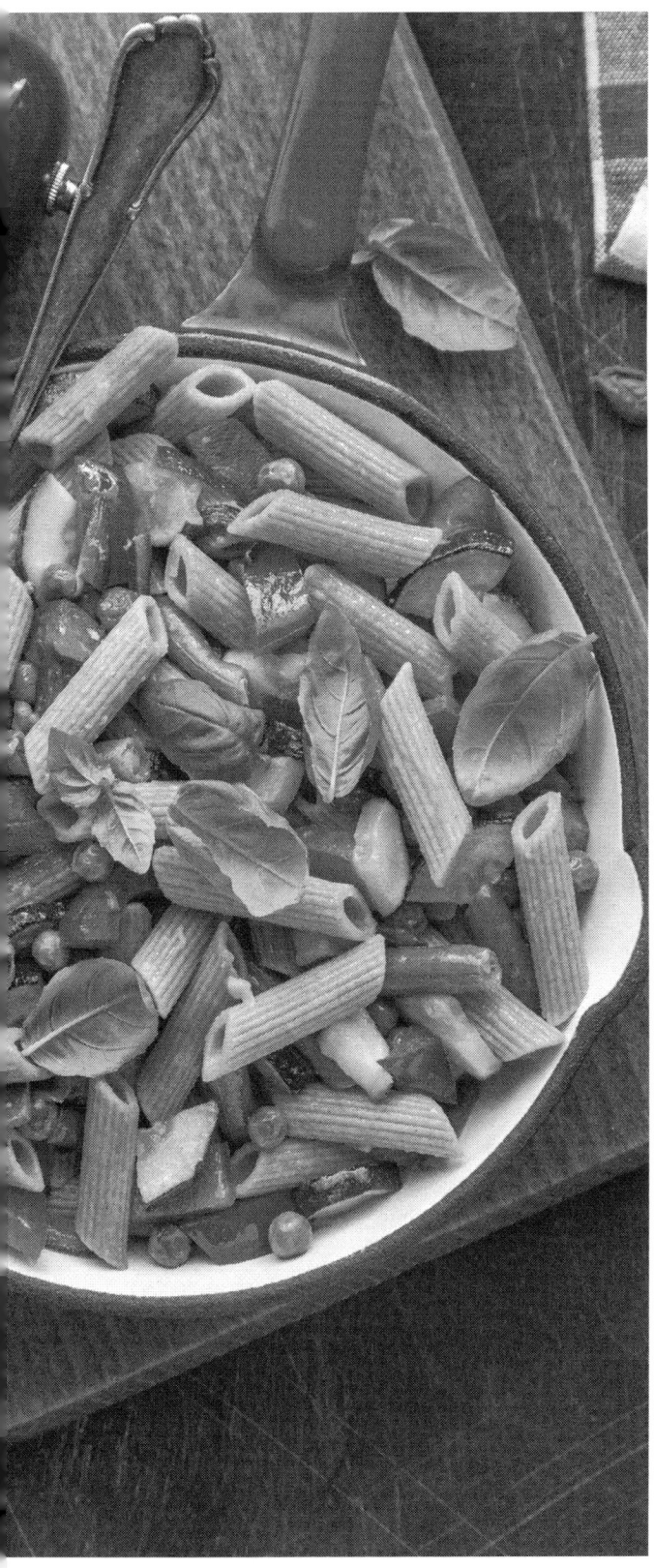

Chickpea And Spinach Cutlets   122

Spinach With Garbanzo Beans   124

Chives Trout   126

Cauliflower Steak With Sweet-Pea Puree   128

Ginger Halibut   130

Tomato Turkey Meatballs   132

Sweet Potato And White Bean Skillet   134

Cabbage And Chicken Mix   136

Spicy Garlic Butter Shrimp   138

Chicken With Pumpkin   140

Chicken & Veggies Tortilla Soup   142

Cashew Turkey Medley   144

Turkey Meatballs With Tomato Sauce   146

SNACKS & DESSERTS   148

Zucchini Dip   150

Delicious Hummus   152

Cauliflower Popcorn   154

Fried Mushrooms   156

Marinated Olives   158

Strawberry & Blueberry Smoothie   160

Rainbow Fruit Salad   162

Kale Dip   164

Coconut Blackberry Smoothie   166

Kale And Almonds   168

CONCLUSION   170

INTRODUCTION

In the labyrinth of dietary approaches, where fads and trends collide, a radiant beacon emerges: the GOLO Diet. It is a resplendent tapestry woven with scientific insight, unveiling a path towards sustainable health and weight management. Embark on this transformative journey and discover a lifestyle that harmonizes with your body, mind, and spirit.

The GOLO Diet is designed for those seeking a holistic approach to weight loss and well-being. It beckons to the weary souls burdened by the shackles of yo-yo dieting, promising liberation from the cycles of deprivation and guilt. Whether you yearn to shed excess pounds, enhance your vitality, or cultivate a deeper understanding of your body, this diet embraces all with open arms.

At the core of the GOLO Diet lies the profound wisdom of insulin regulation. This vital hormone, orchestrator of the body's metabolic symphony, dances delicately upon the tightrope of blood sugar balance. When the scales tip, chaos ensues, and weight gain becomes an unrelenting companion. The GOLO Diet seeks equilibrium, delicately realigning these internal forces, transforming the body into a temple of harmony.

Gone are the days of draconian calorie restrictions and the lament of forbidden foods. The GOLO Diet celebrates the vibrant spectrum of nourishment, encouraging the consumption of nutrient-dense fare that satiates both the palate and the body's deepest cravings. It embraces the embraceable complexities of the human appetite, fostering a sustainable relationship with food that transcends the limitations of mere sustenance.

Enchanting as a moonlit dance, the GOLO Diet orchestrates a symphony of balance, pairing the crescendo of nourishment with the gentle rhythm of physical activity. It beckons you to lace up your shoes, traverse verdant landscapes, and engage in movements that celebrate the body's grace and resilience. Exercise becomes an act of self-expression, an ode to the wonders of the corporeal vessel that propels you forward on your journey.

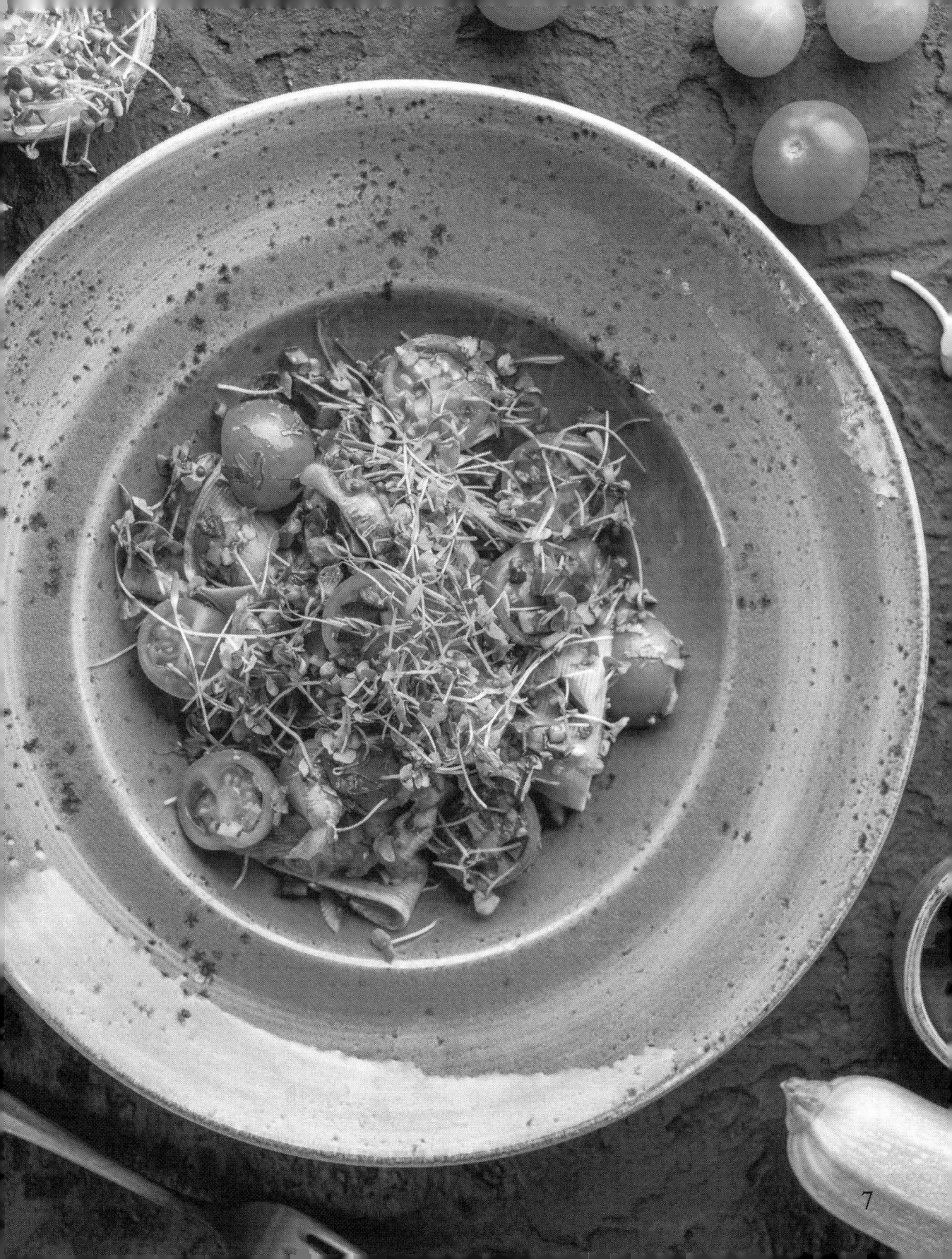

Gone are the days of draconian calorie restrictions and the lament of forbidden foods. The GOLO Diet celebrates the vibrant spectrum of nourishment, encouraging the consumption of nutrient-dense fare that satiates both the palate and the body's deepest cravings. It embraces the embraceable complexities of the human appetite, fostering a sustainable relationship with food that transcends the limitations of mere sustenance.

Enchanting as a moonlit dance, the GOLO Diet orchestrates a symphony of balance, pairing the crescendo of nourishment with the gentle rhythm of physical activity. It beckons you to lace up your shoes, traverse verdant landscapes, and engage in movements that celebrate the body's grace and resilience. Exercise becomes an act of self-expression, an ode to the wonders of the corporeal vessel that propels you forward on your journey.

Immerse yourself in the opulent tapestry of the GOLO Diet, as it guides you through the labyrinth of health, illuminating the path towards sustainable weight loss and vitality. Within these pages, you will find the nourishing principles that underpin this remarkable approach, unlocking the secrets to balanced blood sugar, satiety, and lasting transformation. Embrace the GOLO Diet as a compass, leading you to a destination where self-acceptance, energy, and well-being intertwine.

The symphony of health awaits, and the GOLO Diet invites you to become its maestro. Unleash your potential, embrace your authenticity, and embark on a voyage of self-discovery. Together, we shall unfurl the sails, navigate uncharted waters, and witness the transformative power of the GOLO Diet.

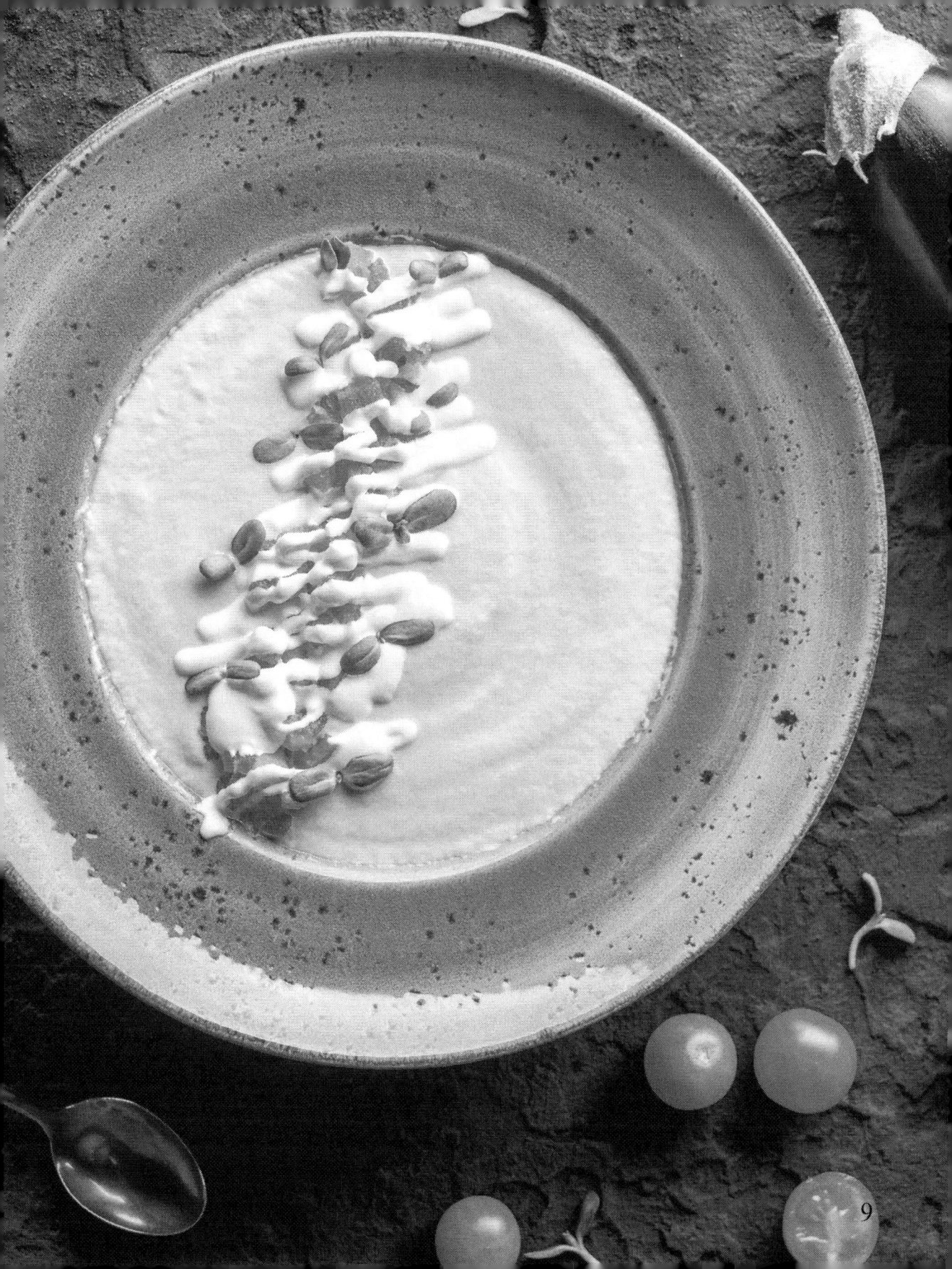

WHAT IS GOLO DIET?

This diet represents a modern and effective approach to weight loss and achieving a healthy lifestyle. GOLO Diet is not just about shedding pounds; it's about transforming your relationship with food, nourishing your body, and optimizing your overall well-being.

At its core, GOLO Diet focuses on regulating insulin levels in the body. Insulin, a hormone secreted by the pancreas, plays a vital role in managing blood sugar levels. When insulin levels are imbalanced, it can lead to weight gain, increased inflammation, and other health complications.

Unlike many fad diets that promote extreme calorie restriction or eliminate entire food groups, GOLO Diet takes a more balanced and sustainable approach. It emphasizes the consumption of nutrient-dense foods that provide essential vitamins, minerals, and antioxidants, while minimizing the intake of processed and sugary foods.

One of the key principles of GOLO Diet is understanding the impact of the Glycemic Index (GI) on your body. The GI measures how quickly carbohydrates in foods are converted into glucose and released into the bloodstream. By choosing foods with a lower GI, you can help regulate your blood sugar levels, reduce insulin spikes, and promote a steady supply of energy throughout the day.

What sets GOLO Diet apart is its holistic approach that encompasses not only nutrition but also exercise, stress management, and emotional well-being. It recognizes that weight loss and overall health are multifaceted, and addressing various aspects of your lifestyle is crucial for long-term success. Remember, this is not just a diet; it's a lifestyle change that will empower you to take control of your health and well-being.

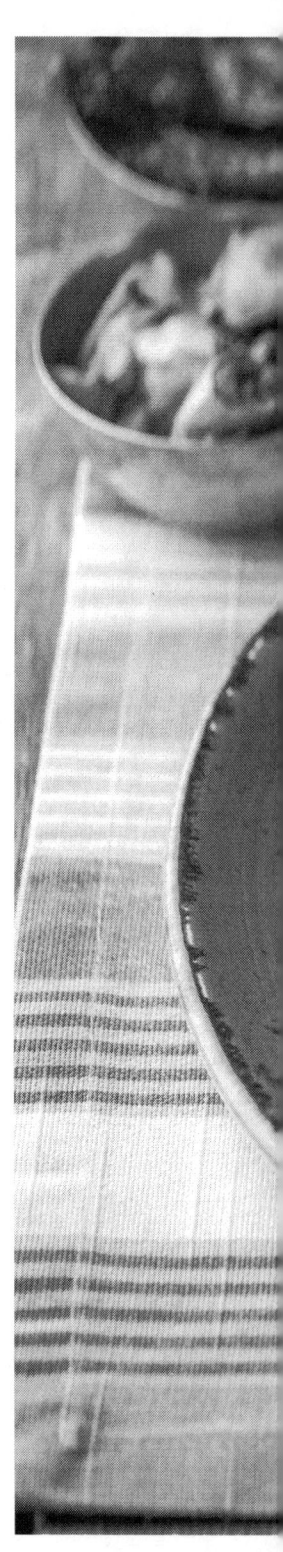

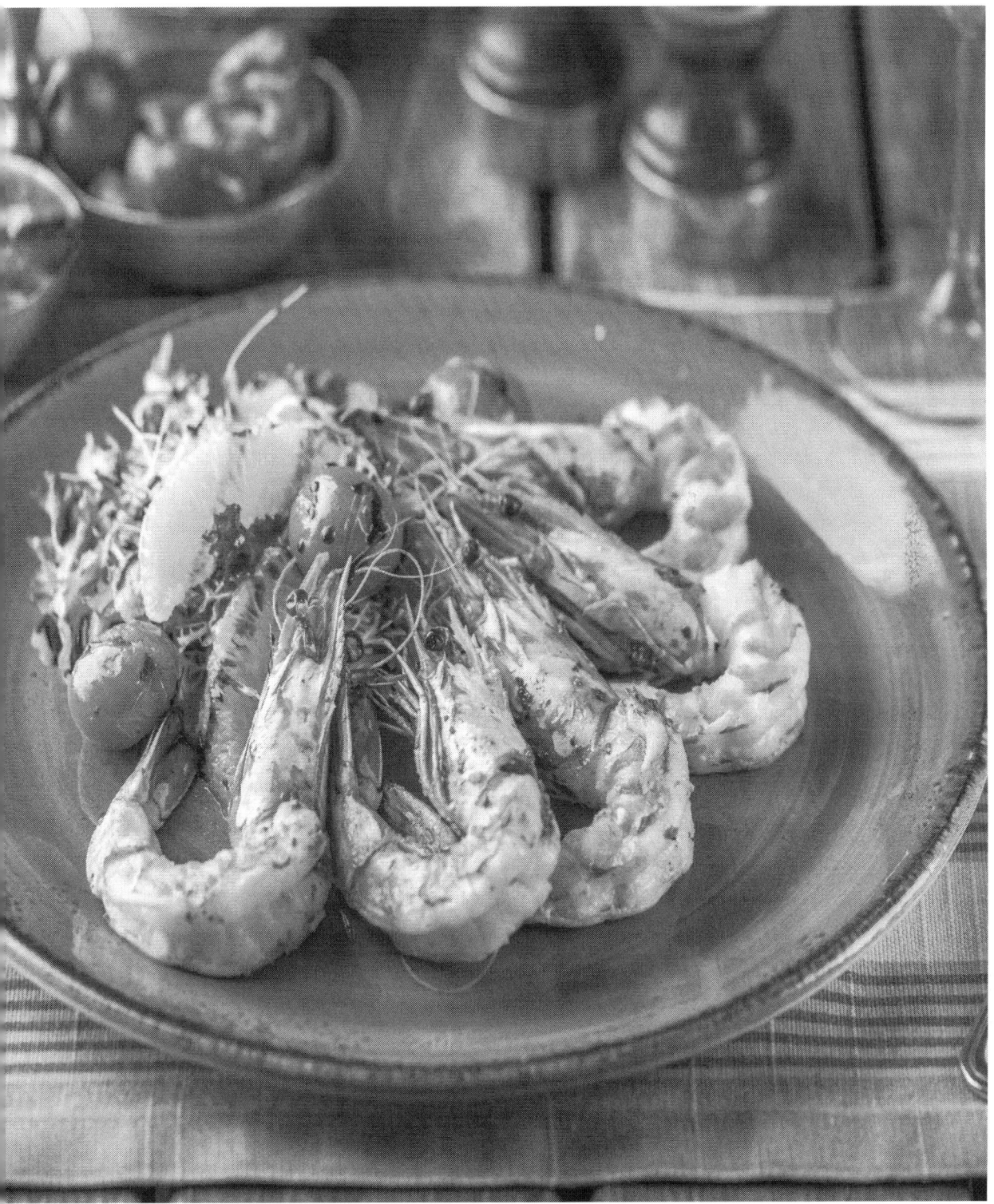

Philosophy Behind The Golo Diet

The philosophy behind the GOLO Diet is grounded in a comprehensive understanding of how our bodies function and the factors that contribute to weight management. At the core of this philosophy is the recognition that insulin, a hormone responsible for regulating blood sugar levels, plays a crucial role in weight gain and overall health.

Unlike traditional diets that focus solely on calorie counting or restrictive eating, the GOLO Diet takes a more nuanced approach. It acknowledges that weight gain is often the result of disrupted insulin levels and aims to restore balance in the body. By addressing the root cause of weight gain, the GOLO Diet offers a sustainable solution for long-term weight management.

Central to the GOLO Diet is the emphasis on eating nutrient-dense, whole foods. These foods provide essential vitamins, minerals, and antioxidants that support overall health and nourish the body. By choosing wholesome options and avoiding processed and sugary foods, individuals can improve their overall well-being and achieve weight loss goals.

Another key aspect of the GOLO Diet is the recognition of the importance of physical activity. Exercise not only helps burn calories but also boosts metabolism and enhances overall fitness. By incorporating regular exercise into their routine, individuals following the GOLO Diet can optimize their weight loss efforts and improve their overall health.

The GOLO Diet also acknowledges the impact of emotions on eating habits and weight management. Emotional eating, stress, and negative self-perceptions can all contribute to weight gain and hinder progress. To address this, the GOLO Diet encourages individuals to develop a mindful approach to their emotions, manage stress effectively, and foster a positive relationship with themselves.

Ultimately, the philosophy behind the GOLO Diet revolves around a holistic understanding of weight management. By addressing the underlying factors that contribute to weight gain—such as insulin regulation, nutrition, exercise, and emotional well-being—the GOLO Diet offers a comprehensive approach to achieving and maintaining a healthy weight.

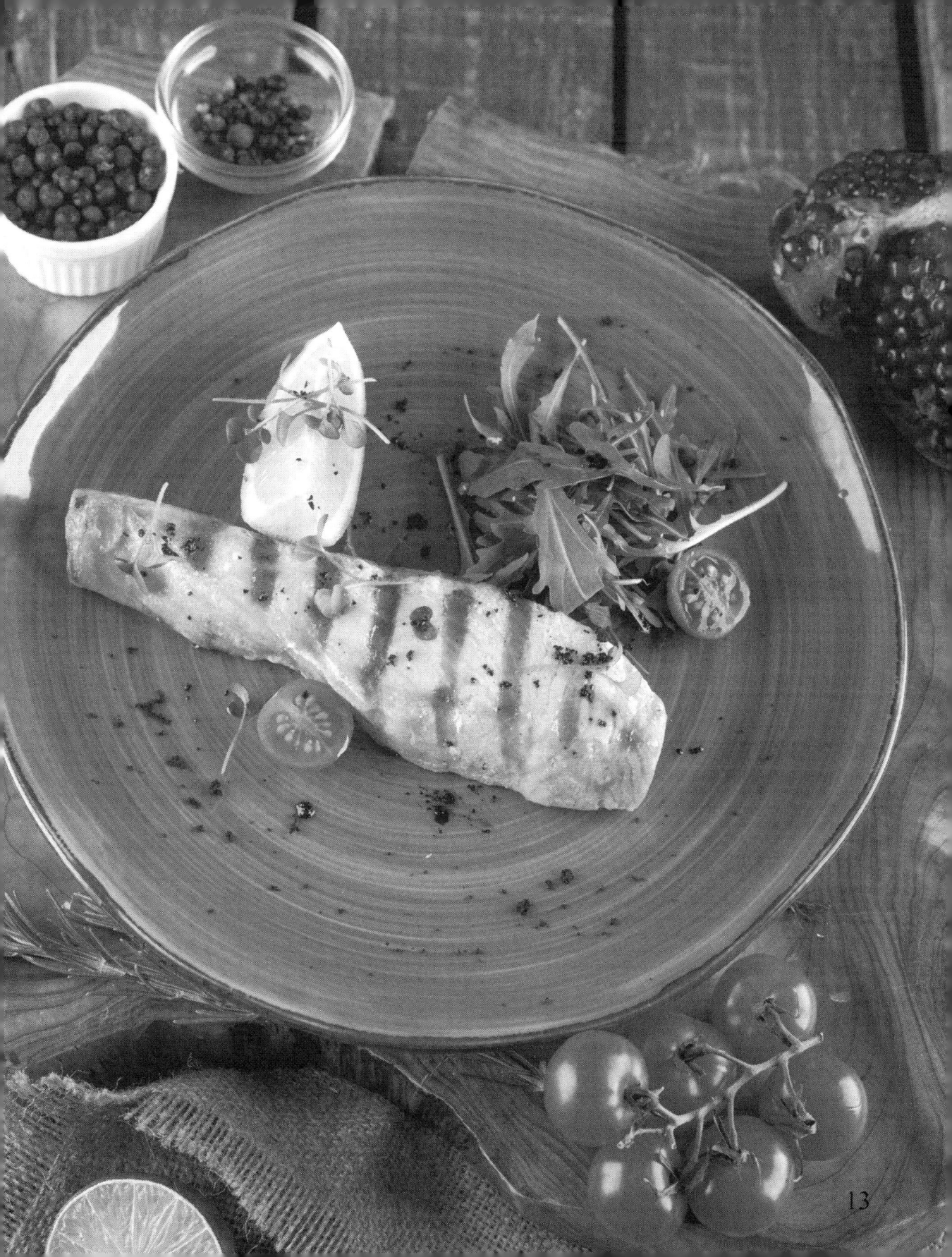

Phases of the GOLO Diet

The GOLO Diet presents a structured approach to weight management, divided into distinct phases that guide individuals towards sustainable and lasting results. These phases provide a roadmap for embracing the principles of the GOLO Diet and achieving optimal health. Let's explore the phases of the GOLO Diet and understand how they contribute to successful weight loss.

Phase 1: Release
The first phase of the GOLO Diet is known as the Release phase. During this phase, individuals focus on balancing their blood sugar levels and jump-starting their metabolism. In the Release phase, individuals typically experience weight loss as their bodies adjust to a healthier eating pattern. This phase helps break the cycle of insulin resistance and establishes a solid foundation for long-term weight management.

Phase 2: Rebalance
After the Release phase comes the Rebalance phase. In this phase, individuals continue to follow the principles of the GOLO Diet but with more flexibility in their food choices. The emphasis remains on consuming nutrient-dense, whole foods and avoiding processed and sugary options.

Phase 3: Reinstate
Once individuals have achieved their weight loss goals, they transition into the Reinstate phase. This phase focuses on maintaining the progress made and embracing the GOLO Diet principles as a way of life. It emphasizes the importance of continued healthy eating, regular exercise, and ongoing support to sustain weight loss and overall well-being.

The phases of the GOLO Diet offer a comprehensive framework for individuals seeking to achieve and maintain a healthy weight. By following the structured approach outlined in each phase, individuals can gradually transform their lifestyle, regulate their insulin levels, and experience long-lasting weight loss and improved overall health.

14

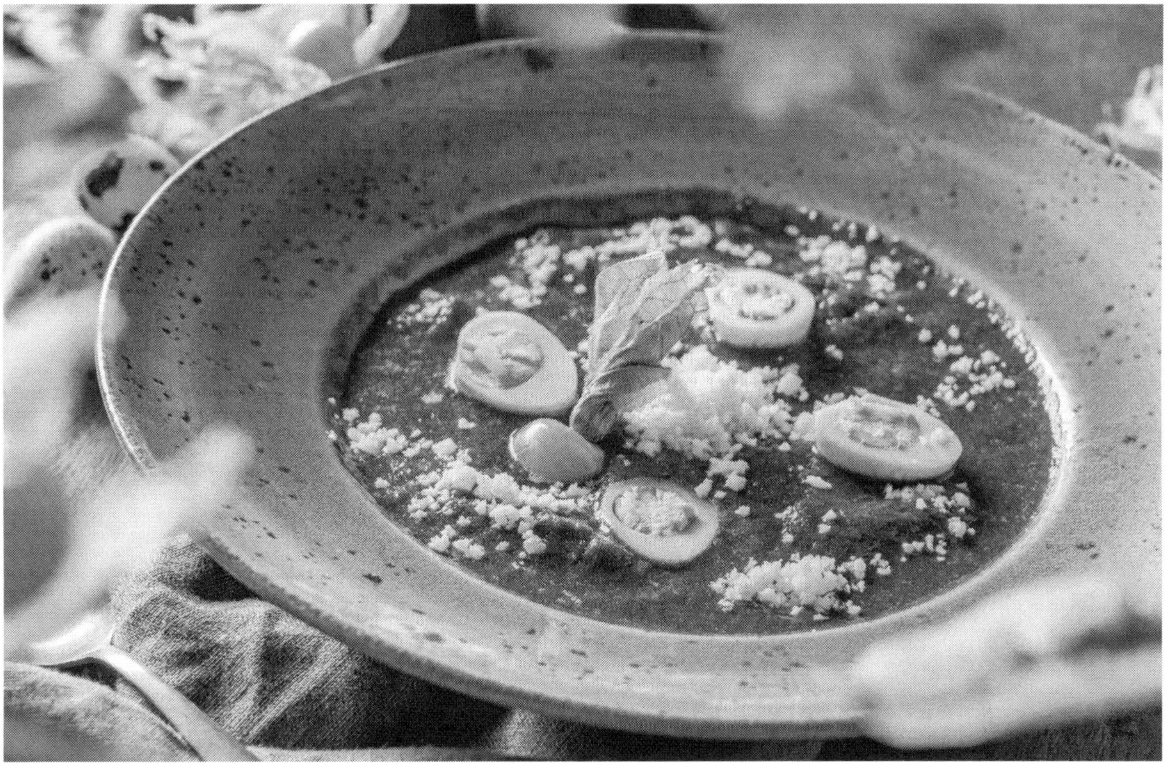

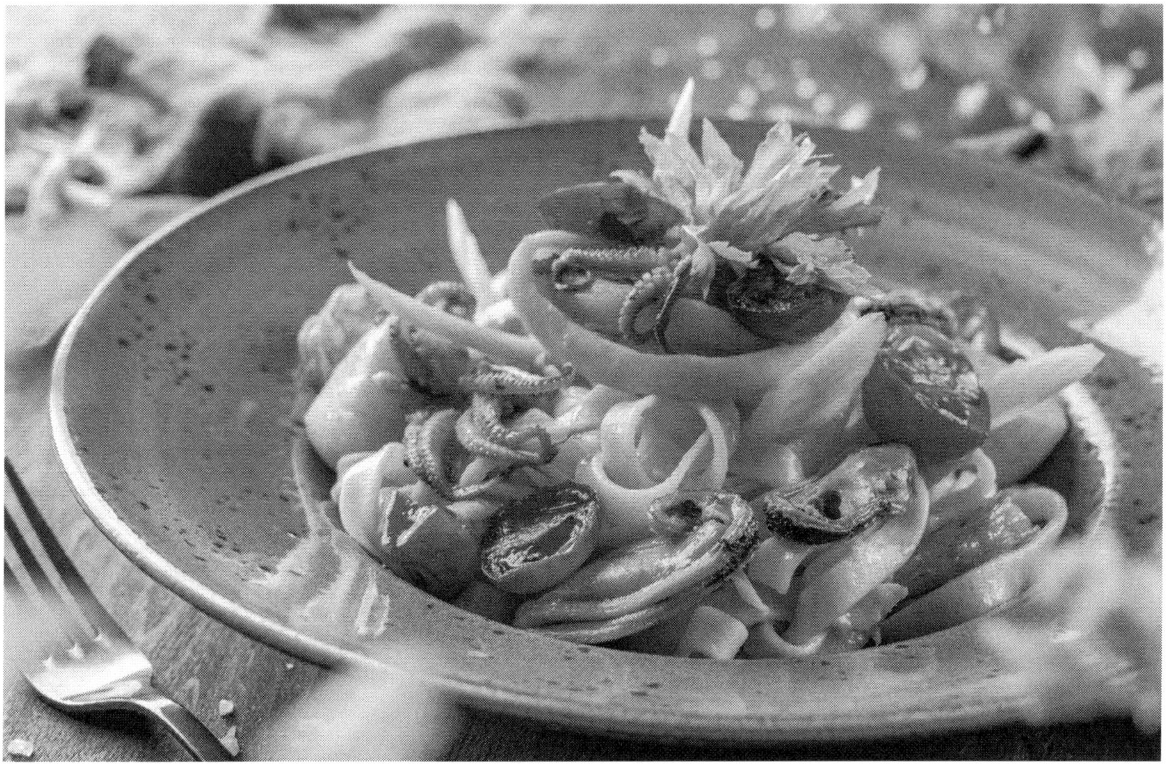

Proper Nutrition and the Glycemic Index

In the quest for optimal health and weight management, understanding the role of proper nutrition and the glycemic index is paramount.

Proper nutrition forms the bedrock of the GOLO Diet. It goes beyond simply counting calories and dives into the quality of the foods we consume. The goal is to nourish our bodies with nutrient-dense, whole foods that provide essential vitamins, minerals, and antioxidants. These foods fuel our bodies, support overall health, and optimize weight loss efforts.

One essential tool in the realm of proper nutrition is the glycemic index (GI). The glycemic index measures how quickly carbohydrates in foods raise blood sugar levels. Foods are assigned a value on a scale from 0 to 100 based on their impact on blood sugar. Low-GI foods, with a value of 55 or less, cause a slower and more gradual rise in blood sugar levels. High-GI foods, with a value of 70 or more, result in a rapid spike in blood sugar.

Choosing foods with a low glycemic index is a key aspect of the GOLO Diet. By incorporating more low-GI foods into your meals, you can maintain balanced blood sugar levels, regulate insulin production, and promote a steady release of energy throughout the day. This helps to prevent cravings, reduce hunger, and support weight loss efforts.

Some examples of low-GI foods include non-starchy vegetables, whole grains, legumes, and certain fruits. These foods are digested and absorbed more slowly, providing a sustained release of energy and promoting feelings of satiety.

On the other hand, high-GI foods, such as processed and refined carbohydrates, sugary snacks, and sugary beverages, can lead to rapid spikes in blood sugar levels. These spikes are often followed by crashes, leaving you feeling hungry, fatigued, and more prone to cravings. By minimizing your consumption of high-GI foods and opting for healthier alternatives, you can maintain a more stable blood sugar level and support your weight loss goals.

While the glycemic index is a valuable tool, it is important to consider the overall quality and balance of your diet. The GOLO Diet encourages a balanced approach to nutrition, combining low-GI foods with lean proteins, healthy fats, and adequate fiber.

16

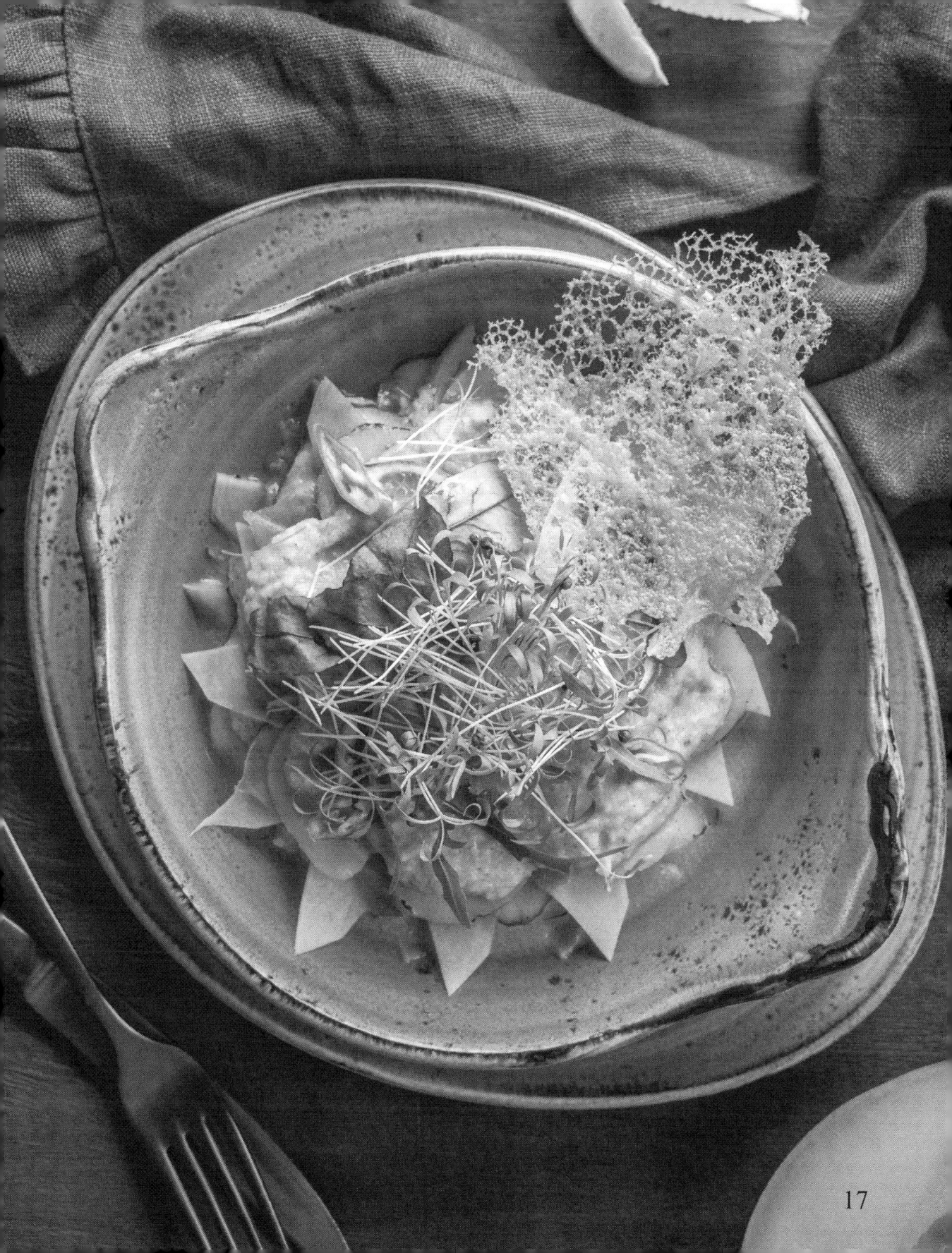

FOODS TO EAT AND AVOID

The GOLO Diet is centered around the idea of consuming nutrient-dense, whole foods that support balanced blood sugar levels, optimize metabolism, and promote sustainable weight loss.

Foods to Eat on the GOLO Diet

Non-Starchy Vegetables:
Fill your plate with an abundance of non-starchy vegetables such as broccoli, spinach, kale, cauliflower, bell peppers, zucchini, and cucumbers. These vegetables are low in calories, high in fiber, and packed with essential vitamins and minerals.

Lean Proteins:
Choose lean sources of protein to fuel your body and support muscle growth and repair. Opt for options such as skinless chicken breast, turkey, fish, tofu, tempeh, legumes (beans, lentils), and Greek yogurt. These protein sources provide essential amino acids while keeping saturated fats in check.

Whole Grains:
Incorporate whole grains into your diet for sustained energy and fiber. Include options like quinoa, brown rice, whole wheat bread and pasta, oats, barley, and bulgur. These whole grains are nutrient-rich and help regulate blood sugar levels.

Healthy Fats:
Embrace the power of healthy fats, which play a vital role in satiety and overall well-being. Include sources like avocados, nuts (almonds, walnuts, pistachios), seeds (chia seeds, flaxseeds), olive oil, and fatty fish (salmon, mackerel). These fats provide essential omega-3 fatty acids and promote heart health.

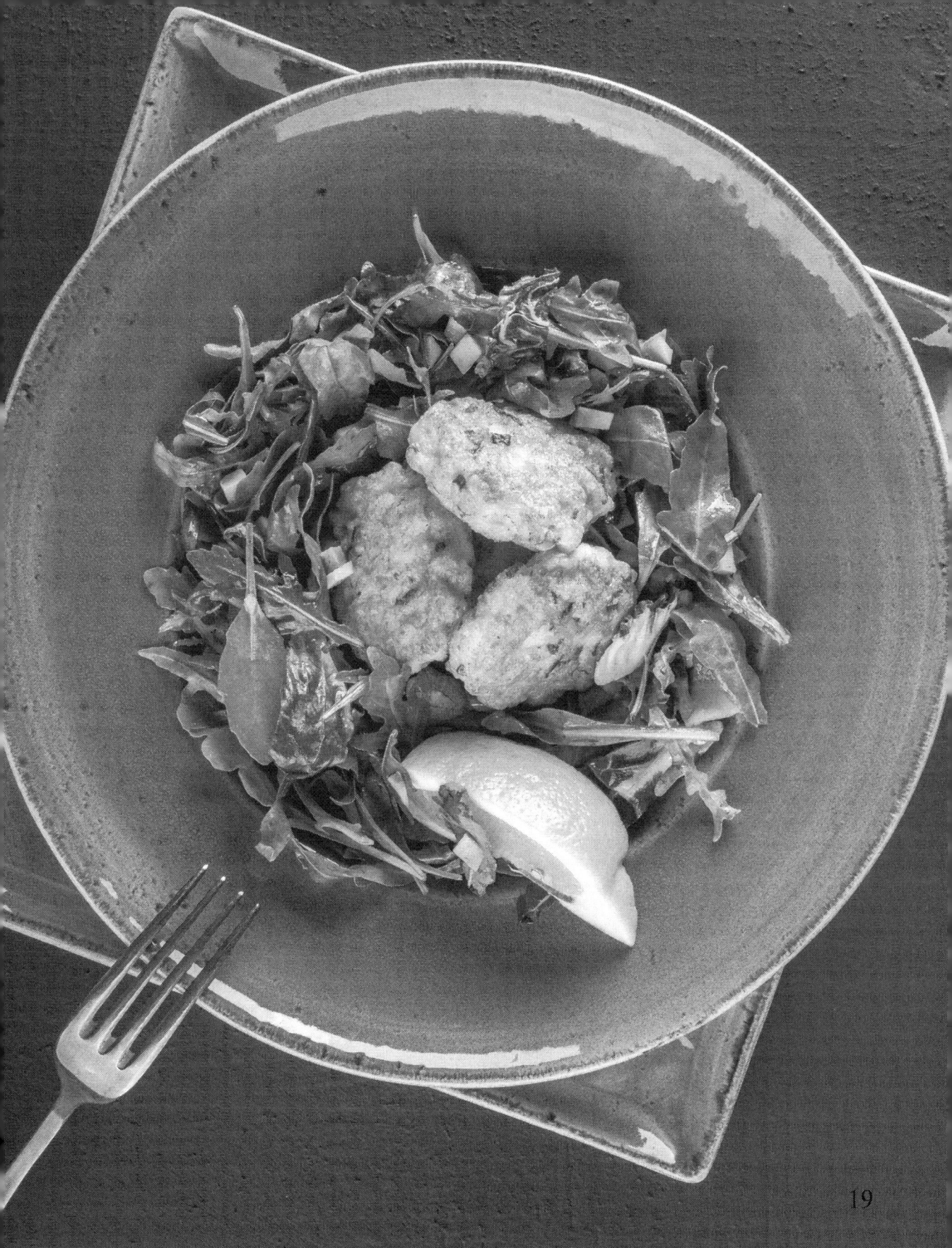

Low-Glycemic Fruits:
Enjoy a variety of fruits that have a lower impact on blood sugar levels. Opt for options like berries (strawberries, blueberries, raspberries), apples, pears, citrus fruits (oranges, grapefruits), and cherries. These fruits provide natural sweetness and valuable nutrients.

Dairy or Dairy Alternatives:
Incorporate low-fat dairy or dairy alternatives into your diet for calcium and protein. Choose options such as skim milk, unsweetened almond milk, Greek yogurt, and cottage cheese. Be mindful of added sugars in flavored varieties.

Herbs, Spices, and Flavor Enhancers:
Enhance the taste of your meals with herbs, spices, and flavor enhancers like garlic, ginger, turmeric, cinnamon, cayenne pepper, and vinegar. These additions provide depth and character to your dishes without adding unnecessary calories.

Hydration:
Stay hydrated by drinking plenty of water throughout the day. Water is essential for maintaining overall health and supporting weight loss efforts. You can also enjoy herbal teas and unsweetened beverages as alternatives.

Remember, portion control is a key aspect of the GOLO Diet. Pay attention to your body's hunger and fullness cues, and strive for balanced meals that include a combination of proteins, whole grains, and vegetables. It's important to personalize your meal plan based on your individual preferences, dietary needs, and any specific health considerations.

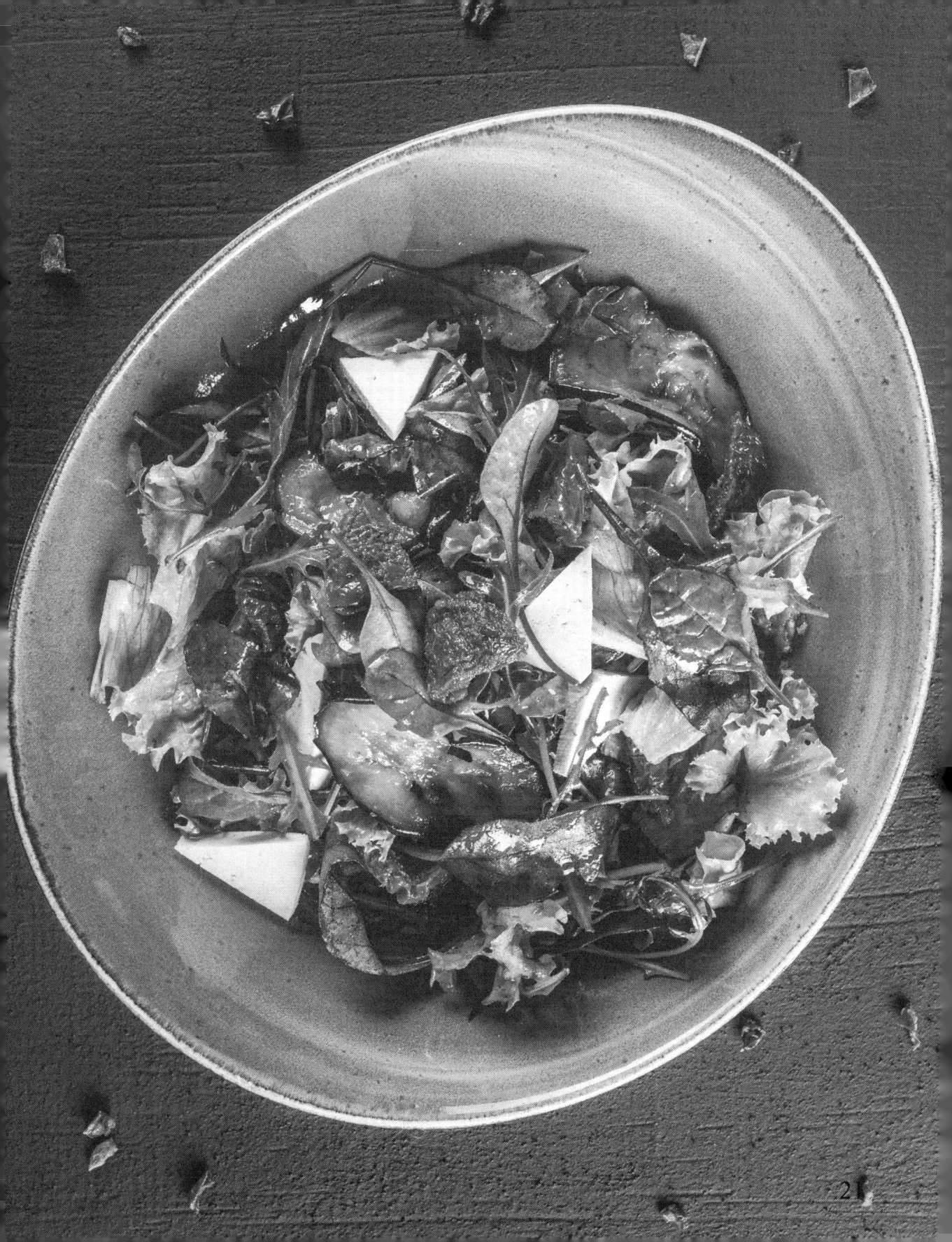

Foods to Avoid on the GOLO Diet

Processed and Refined Carbohydrates:
Steer clear of processed and refined carbohydrates such as white bread, white rice, sugary cereals, pastries, cookies, cakes, and sugary snacks. These foods are typically high in added sugars, devoid of nutrients, and can cause rapid spikes in blood sugar levels.

Sugary Beverages:
Avoid sugary beverages like soda, fruit juices, sweetened tea or coffee drinks, and energy drinks. These beverages are often loaded with added sugars and can lead to significant fluctuations in blood sugar levels.

High-Sugar Foods:
Minimize your consumption of high-sugar foods, including candy, chocolates, ice cream, sweetened yogurts, and sugary condiments. These foods provide empty calories, contribute to cravings, and can sabotage your weight loss efforts.

Processed Meats:
Limit your intake of processed meats, such as sausages, hot dogs, bacon, and deli meats. These meats often contain additives, preservatives, and high amounts of sodium, which may negatively impact your health and weight management goals.

Trans Fats:
Avoid foods high in trans fats, which are typically found in fried foods, packaged snacks, commercially baked goods, and margarine. Trans fats are known to increase the risk of heart disease and can hinder weight loss efforts.

High-Sodium Foods:
Reduce your consumption of high-sodium foods, including salty snacks, canned soups, processed sauces, and fast food. Excess sodium can lead to water retention and bloating, and it is generally recommended to limit sodium intake for overall health.

Sweetened Condiments and Sauces:
Be mindful of condiments and sauces that contain added sugars, such as ketchup, barbecue sauce, salad dressings, and sweetened marinades. Opt for healthier alternatives or make your own versions using natural ingredients.

Alcohol:
While the occasional moderate consumption of alcohol may be permissible for some, it is generally recommended to limit alcohol intake on the GOLO Diet. Alcoholic beverages can contribute to excess calorie consumption, disrupt blood sugar levels, and hinder weight loss progress.

By avoiding these foods on the GOLO Diet, you can minimize the negative impact on insulin levels, stabilize blood sugar, and promote sustainable weight loss. Remember that adopting a balanced and mindful approach to eating is key. Focus on nourishing your body with nutrient-dense, whole foods that support your overall health and well-being.

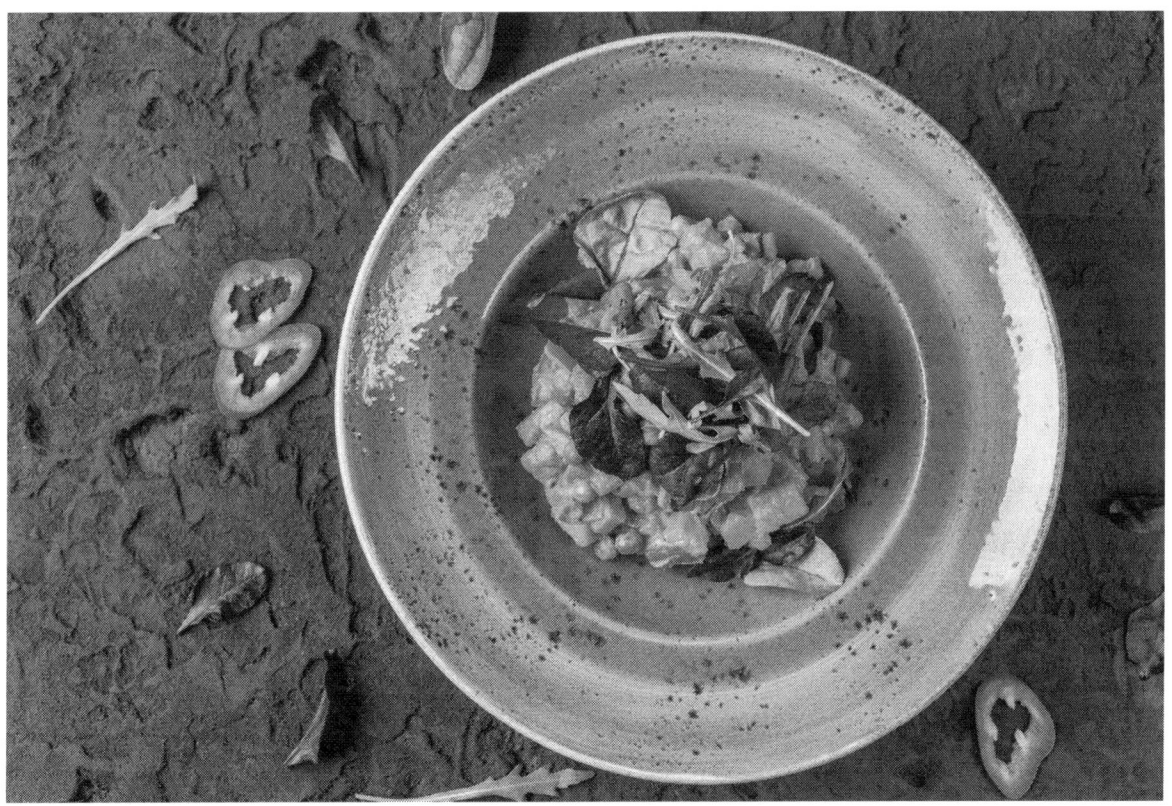

HEALTH BENEFITS GOLO DIET

The GOLO Diet not only supports weight loss but also offers a range of health benefits that can positively impact your overall well-being. This chapter explores the various ways in which the GOLO Diet can enhance your health, promoting not just a slimmer waistline but also improved vitality and long-term wellness.

Balanced Blood Sugar Levels:
The core principle of the GOLO Diet revolves around balancing blood sugar levels. By consuming nutrient-dense foods with a low glycemic index, you can prevent spikes and crashes in blood sugar, reducing the risk of insulin resistance and type 2 diabetes.

Weight Loss and Maintenance:
One of the primary goals of the GOLO Diet is sustainable weight loss. By adopting a structured meal plan that combines whole foods, portion control, and balanced nutrition, individuals can achieve their weight loss goals while maintaining muscle mass. This promotes a healthier body composition and helps to sustain weight loss in the long term.

Improved Cardiovascular Health:
The GOLO Diet emphasizes the consumption of heart-healthy foods, such as lean proteins, whole grains, and healthy fats. These dietary choices, combined with weight loss and balanced blood sugar levels, can reduce the risk of cardiovascular diseases like heart disease and hypertension. Additionally, the inclusion of fiber-rich foods supports healthy cholesterol levels.

Enhanced Energy and Vitality:
By following the GOLO Diet and stabilizing blood sugar levels, you can experience a consistent and sustained release of energy throughout the day. This helps combat fatigue, promotes mental clarity, and improves overall productivity. Steady energy levels also support regular exercise and physical activity, contributing to a more active lifestyle.

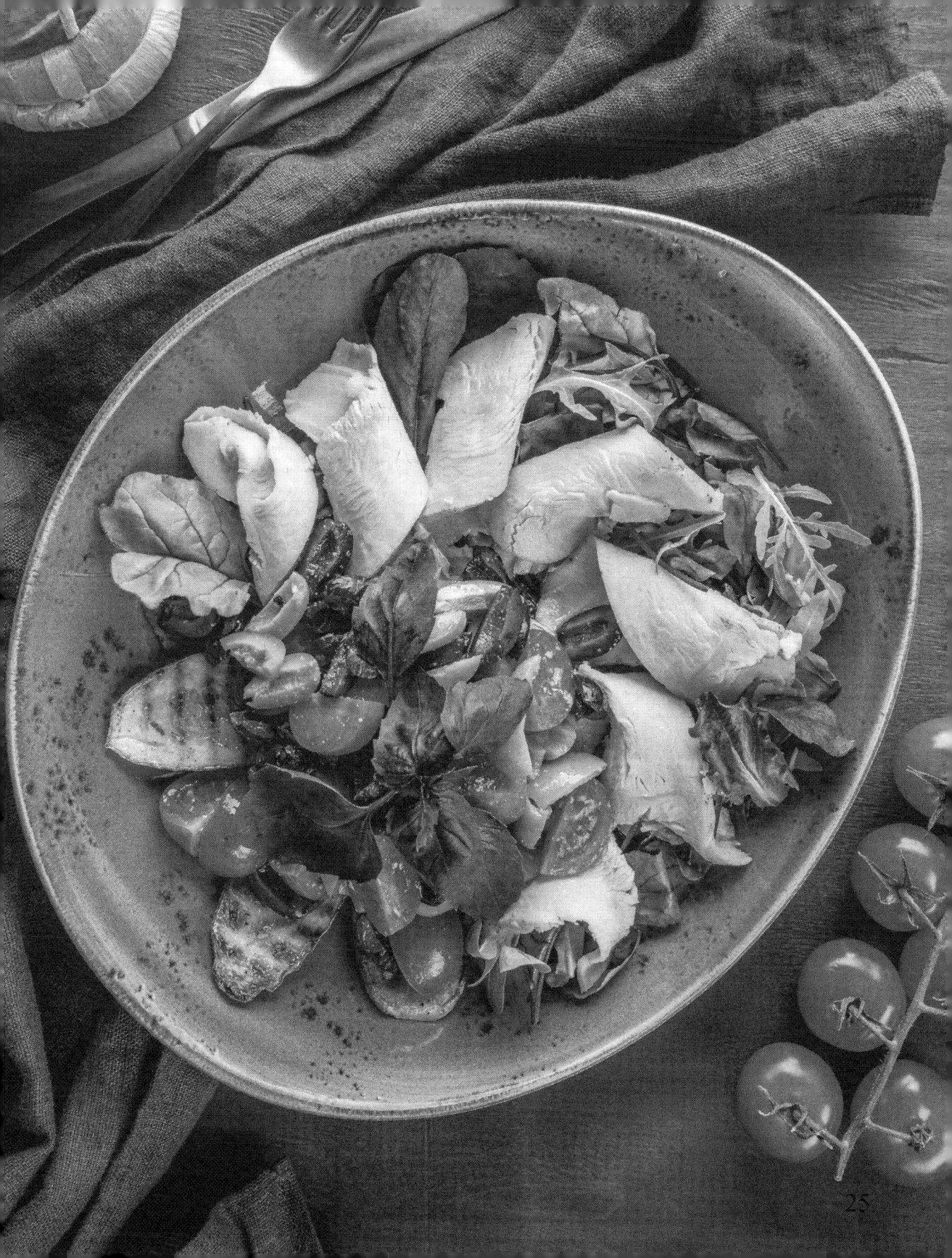

Reduced Inflammation:

The GOLO Diet emphasizes the consumption of whole, unprocessed foods that are rich in antioxidants and anti-inflammatory compounds. By reducing the intake of processed and sugary foods that can contribute to inflammation, individuals on the GOLO Diet may experience a reduction in chronic inflammation, which is linked to various health issues, including obesity, diabetes, and cardiovascular diseases.

Support for Digestive Health:

The GOLO Diet promotes the consumption of fiber-rich foods, including non-starchy vegetables, whole grains, and legumes. These foods support digestive health by promoting regular bowel movements, preventing constipation, and supporting a healthy gut microbiome. A well-functioning digestive system is essential for nutrient absorption, immune function, and overall wellness.

Positive Psychological Impact:

The GOLO Diet focuses on balanced nutrition and mindful eating, encouraging individuals to develop a healthier relationship with food. This can lead to improved mental well-being, increased self-awareness, and reduced emotional eating habits. By nourishing the body with wholesome foods, individuals may experience improved mood, reduced stress levels, and increased self-confidence.

By embracing the GOLO Diet and its principles, you can achieve not only weight loss but also a multitude of health benefits. From balanced blood sugar levels and improved cardiovascular health to increased energy and reduced inflammation, this diet offers a holistic approach to well-being. The combination of nourishing foods, portion control, and mindful eating sets the foundation for a healthier lifestyle that supports long-term vitality and overall wellness.

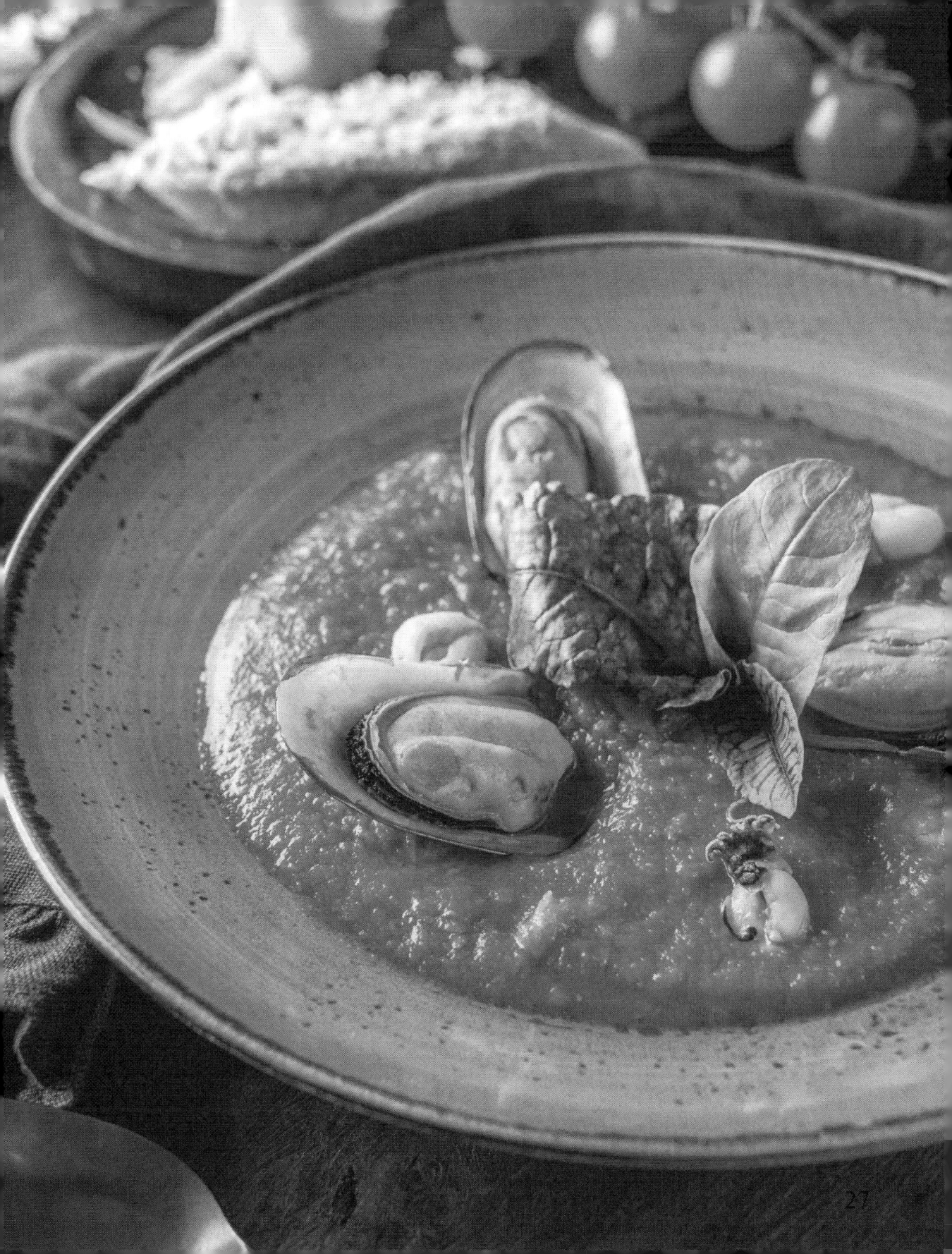

GOLO DIET AND WEIGHT LOSS

This chapter explores how the GOLO Diet can effectively support your weight loss goals and provide you with the tools to make lasting lifestyle changes.

Balanced Blood Sugar Levels for Weight Management:
The foundation of the GOLO Diet lies in stabilizing blood sugar levels. This balanced approach to blood sugar regulation helps you maintain a caloric deficit, a key factor in weight loss.

Portion Control and Balanced Nutrition:
The GOLO Diet emphasizes portion control, ensuring that you consume the right amount of calories for your body's needs. It encourages a balanced combination of lean proteins, complex carbohydrates, and healthy fats, providing essential nutrients while promoting satiety and preventing excessive calorie intake. By learning to listen to your body's hunger and fullness cues, you can achieve a sustainable and healthy rate of weight loss.

Metabolism Optimization:
The GOLO Diet aims to optimize your metabolism, the process by which your body converts food into energy. By nourishing your body with nutrient-dense foods and maintaining balanced blood sugar levels, you can support a healthy metabolism. This can help prevent metabolic slowdown often associated with restrictive diets, enabling more efficient calorie burning and facilitating weight loss.

Supportive Lifestyle Changes:
The GOLO Diet goes beyond a short-term weight loss plan by promoting sustainable lifestyle changes. It encourages regular physical activity, such as exercise and daily movement, to boost calorie burning, improve cardiovascular health, and enhance overall well-being. Additionally, the diet emphasizes mindfulness and self-care practices, fostering a holistic approach to weight management.

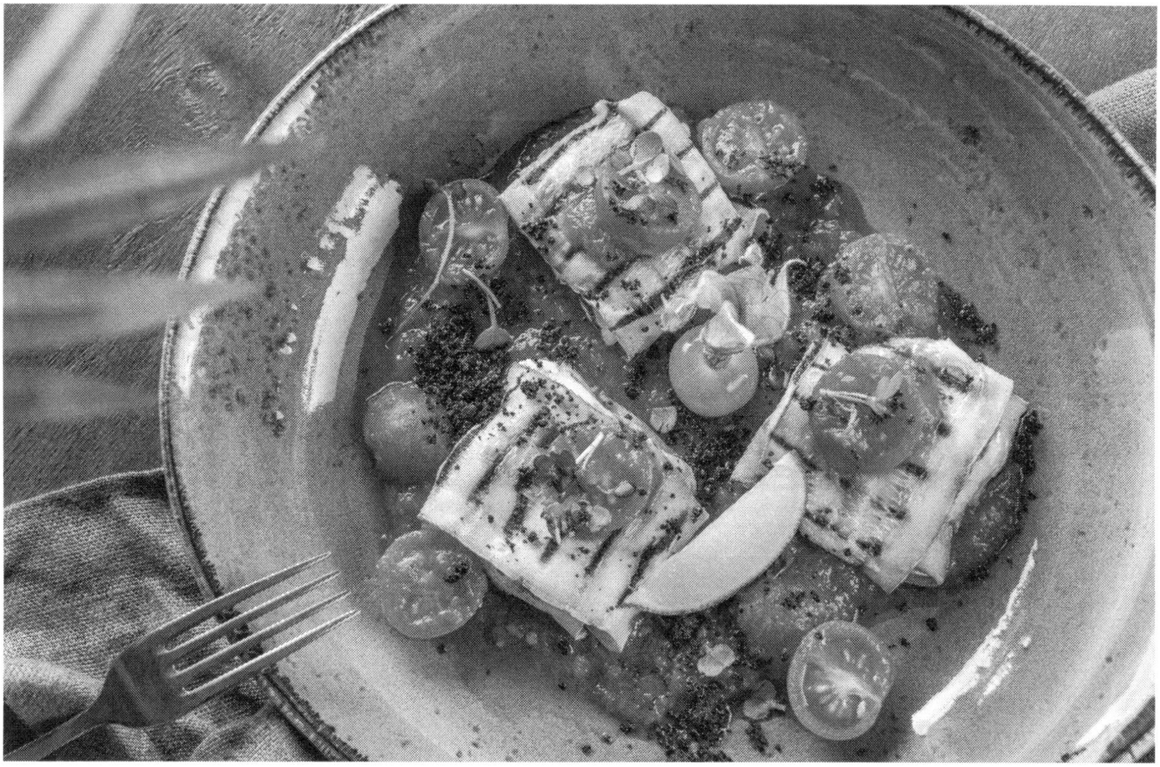

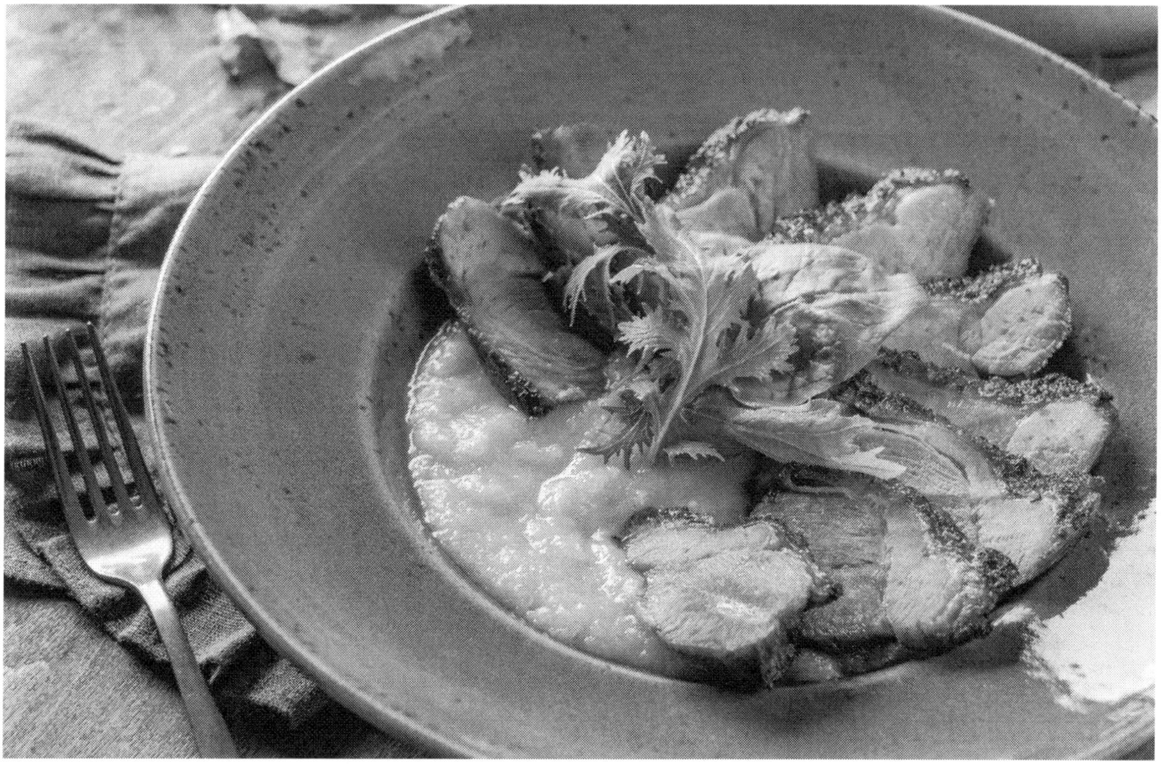

Long-Term Weight Maintenance:
The GOLO Diet equips you with the knowledge and tools needed to maintain your weight loss achievements in the long term. By adopting healthy eating habits, portion control, and balanced nutrition as a lifestyle, you can avoid the pitfalls of yo-yo dieting and weight regain. The emphasis on overall health and well-being sets the stage for sustained weight maintenance and continued progress.

Individualized Approach:
The GOLO Diet recognizes that each person is unique, with different dietary needs, preferences, and goals. It offers flexibility and customization, allowing you to tailor the diet to suit your specific requirements. This individualized approach enhances adherence and increases the likelihood of successful weight loss outcomes.

While the GOLO Diet provides a structured framework for weight loss, it's important to remember that individual results may vary. Factors such as starting weight, overall health, adherence to the diet, and lifestyle choices all play a role in the rate and extent of weight loss. It's essential to consult with a healthcare professional or registered dietitian before embarking on any significant dietary changes.

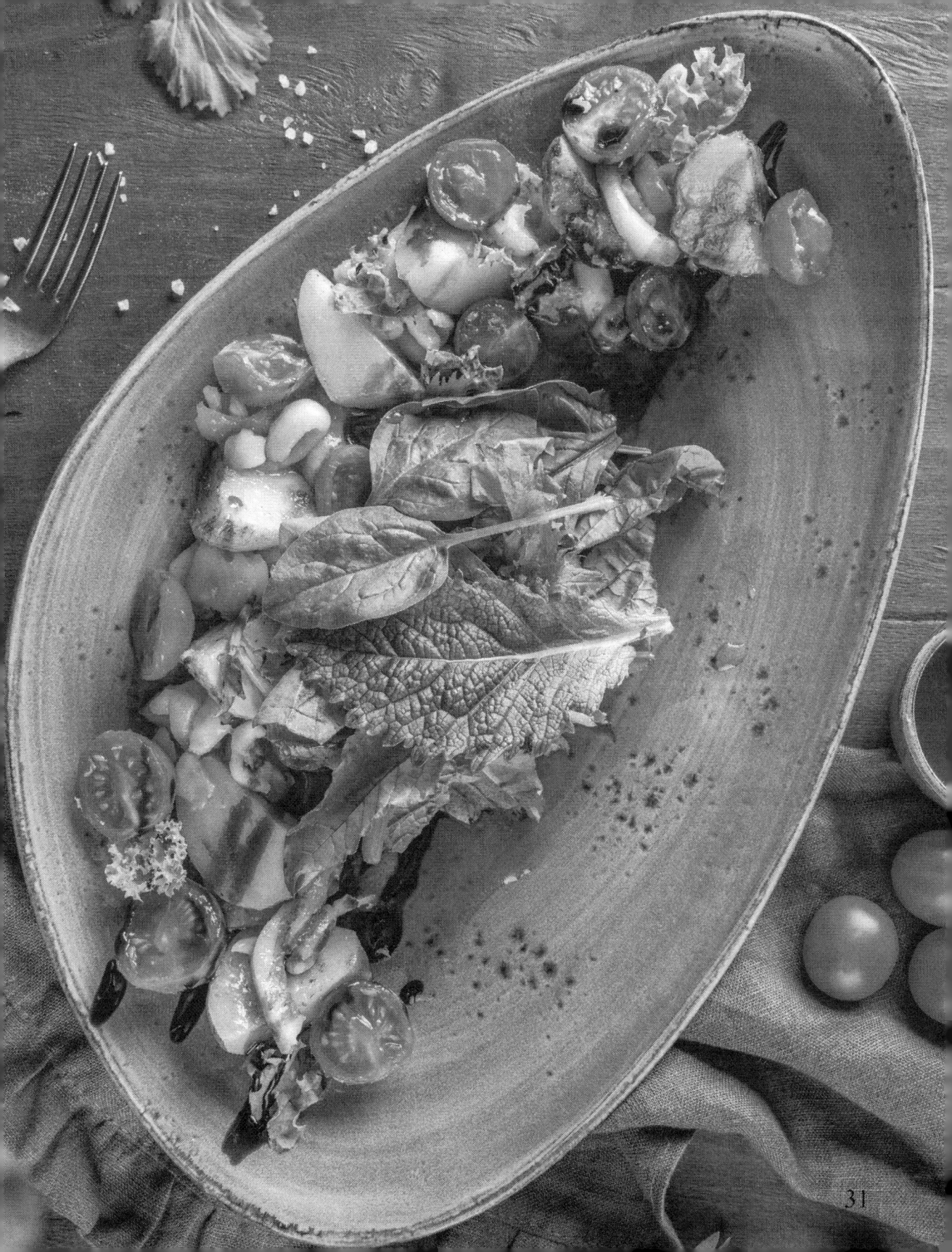

BREAKFAST RECIPES

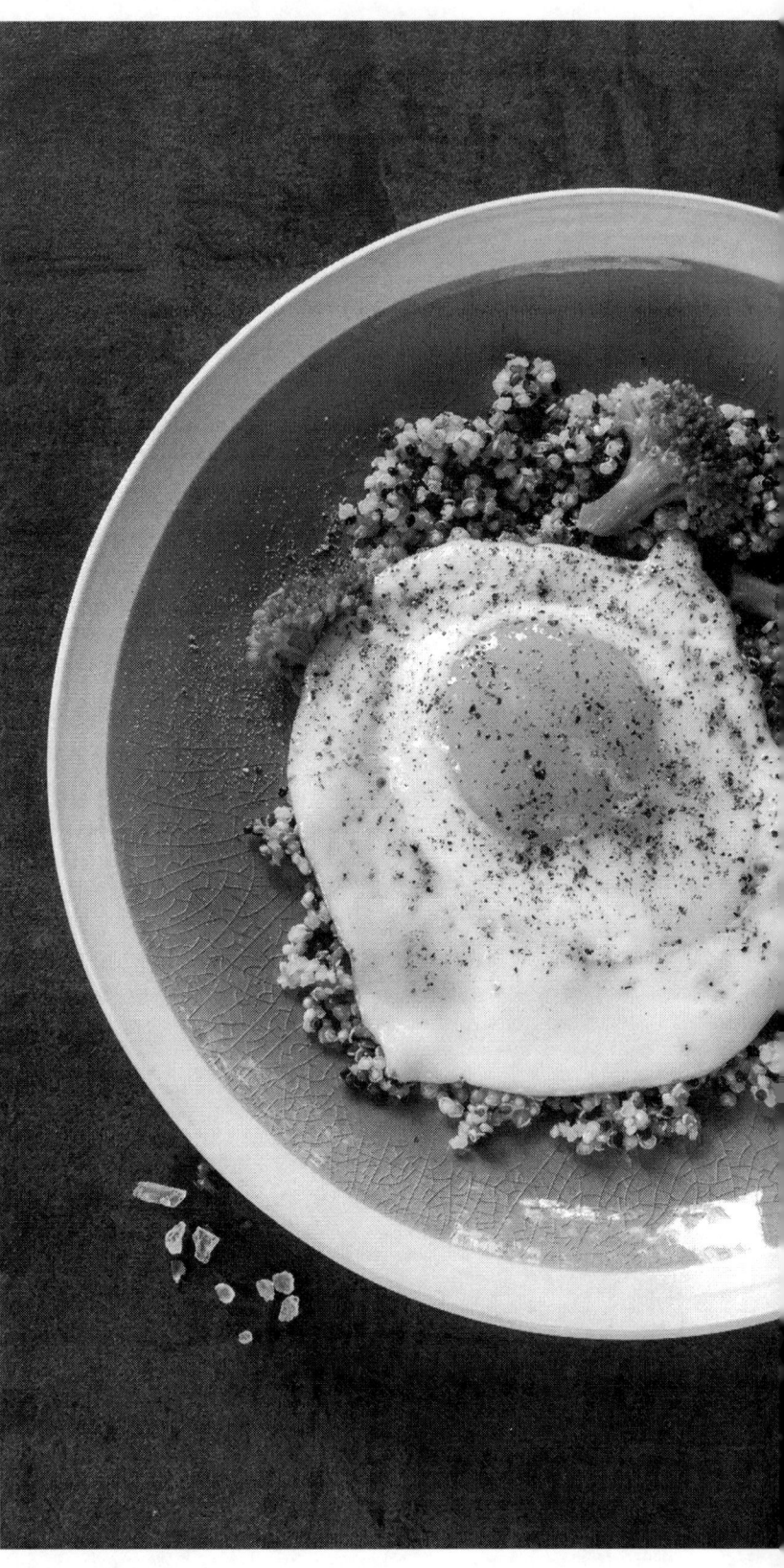

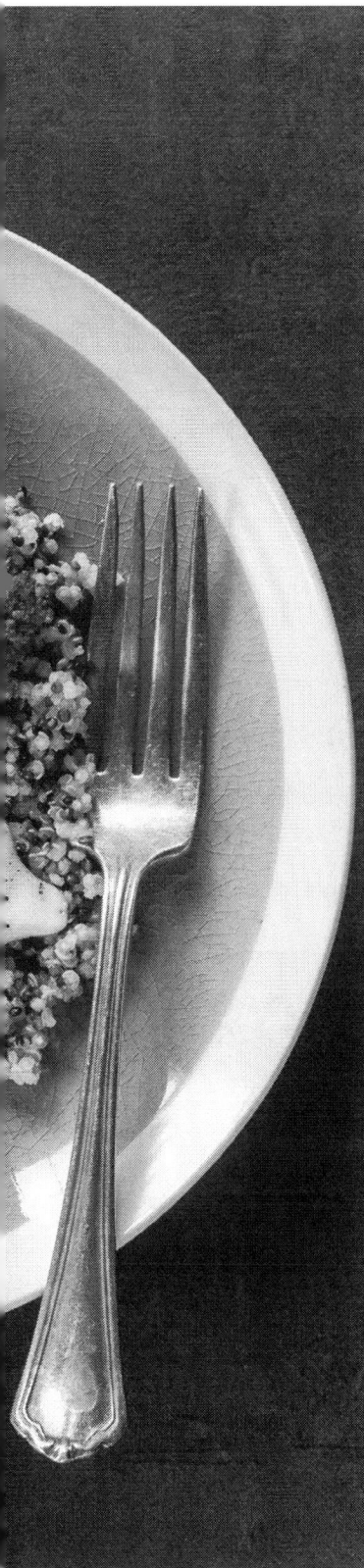

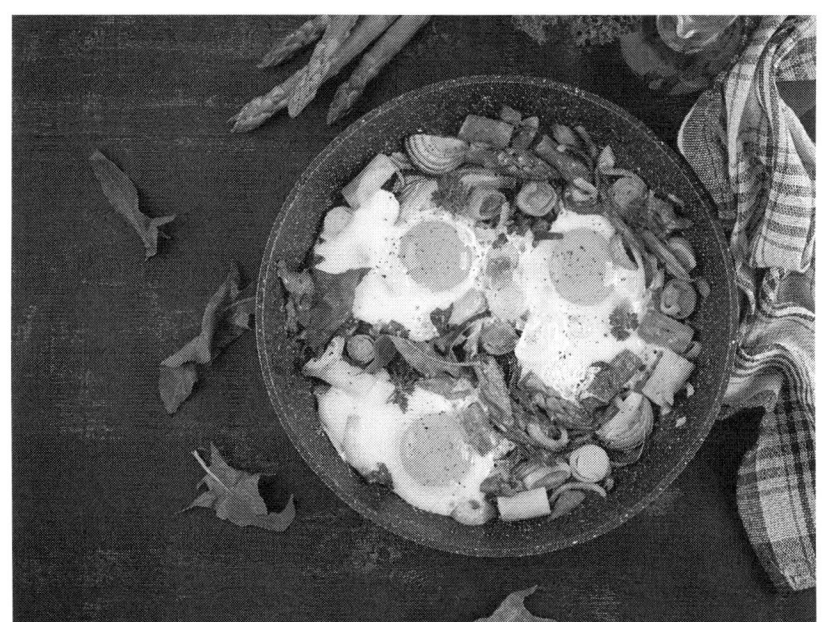

Recipes include foods recommended in the GOLO diet, such as lean sources of protein, lean dairy products, low glycemic index vegetables, whole grains, and healthy sources of fat. Recipes include low to medium GI ingredients to help maintain stable blood sugar levels.

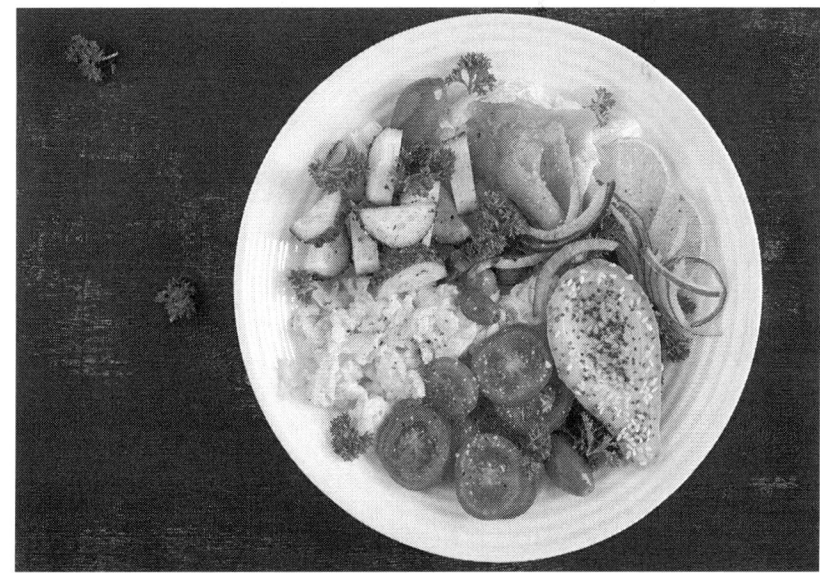

SPINACH OMELET

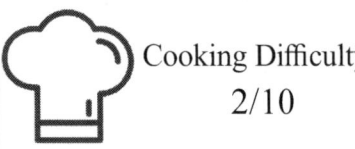 Cooking Difficulty: 2/10	 Cooking Time: 20 minutes	 Servings: 3

INGREDIENTS

- 6 whisked eggs
- 1 c. baby spinach
- black pepper
- 1 tbsp. olive oil
- 2 chopped spring onions
- 1 tsp. sweet paprika

DESCRIPTION

STEP 1

Ensure that you heat the pan; add the spring onions, and paprika, stir, and sauté for 5 minutes.

STEP 2

Add the eggs, spinach, and pepper toss spread into the pan, cover it then cook for 15 minutes. Divide everything between plates and serve.

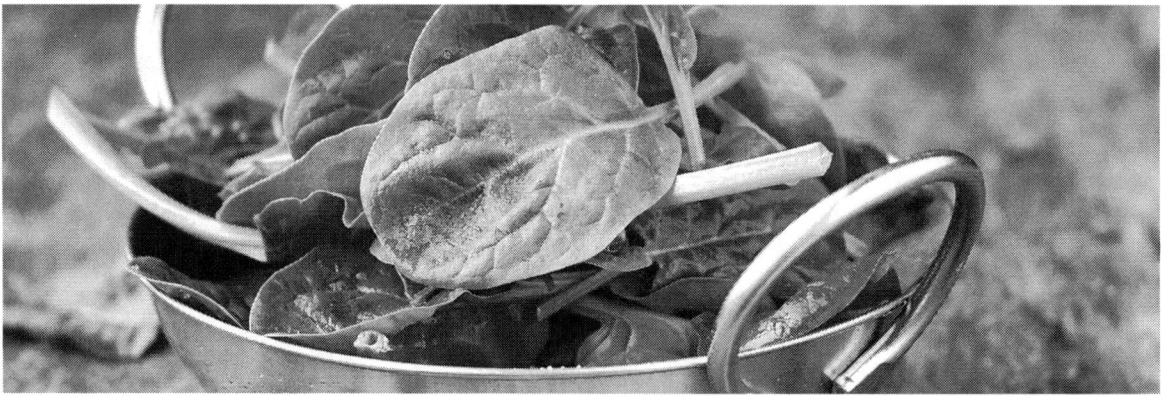

NUTRITIONAL INFORMATION

Calories 245, Fat 7g, Carbs 6g, Protein 9.3g

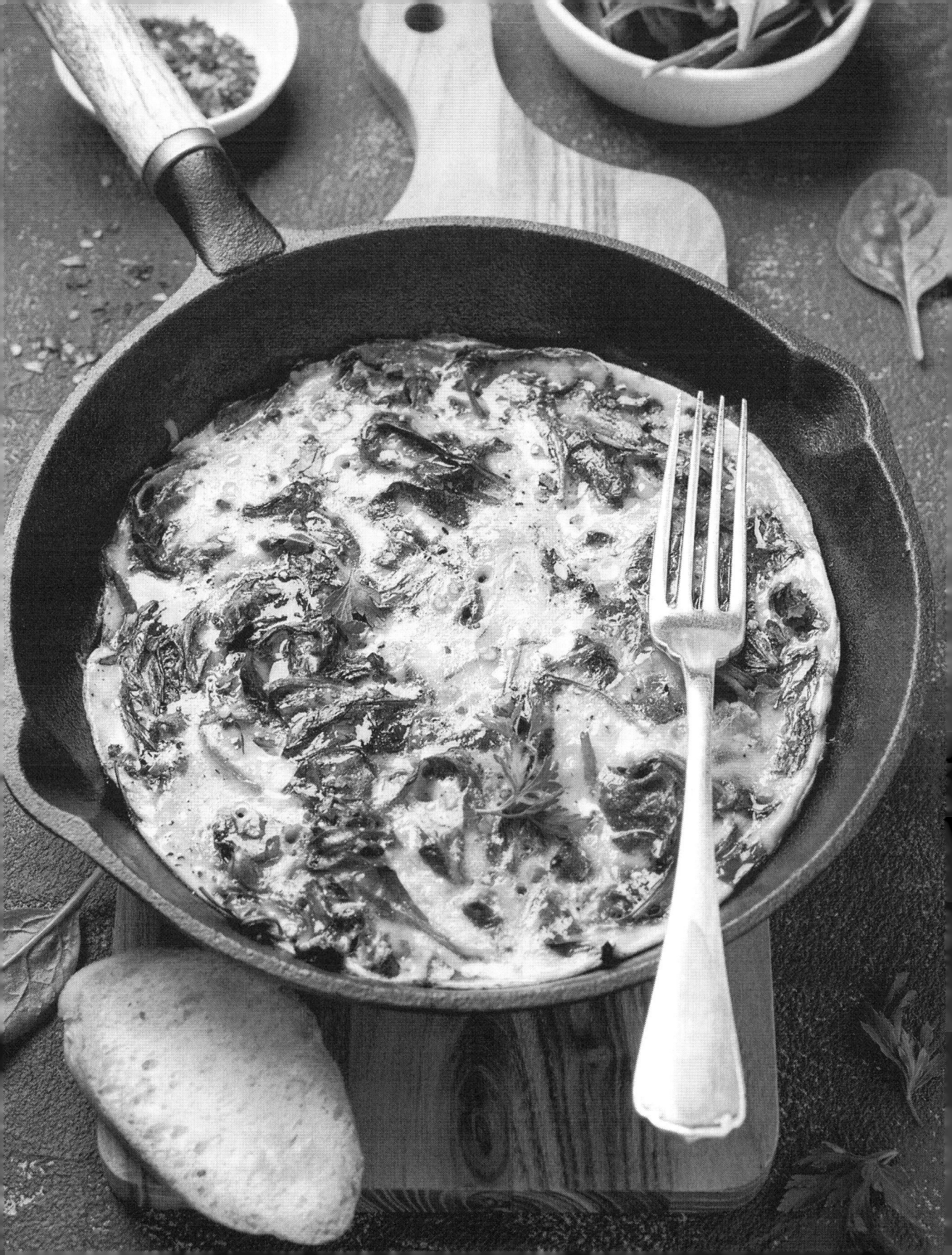

TOMATO AND EGGS SALAD

 Cooking Difficulty: 1/10

 Cooking Time: 3 minutes

 Servings: 4

INGREDIENTS

- 4 hard-boiled eggs, peeled and chopped
- 2 c. halved cherry tomatoes
- 1 c. pitted kalamata olives halved
- 1 c. baby spinach
- 2 chopped spring onions
- black pepper
- 1 tbsp. olive oil

DESCRIPTION

STEP 1
In a salad bowl, combine the tomatoes with the eggs and the other ingredients, toss, divide into smaller bowls and serve for breakfast.

NUTRITIONAL INFORMATION

Calories 126, Fat 5.6g, Carbs 4.9g, Protein 4.9g

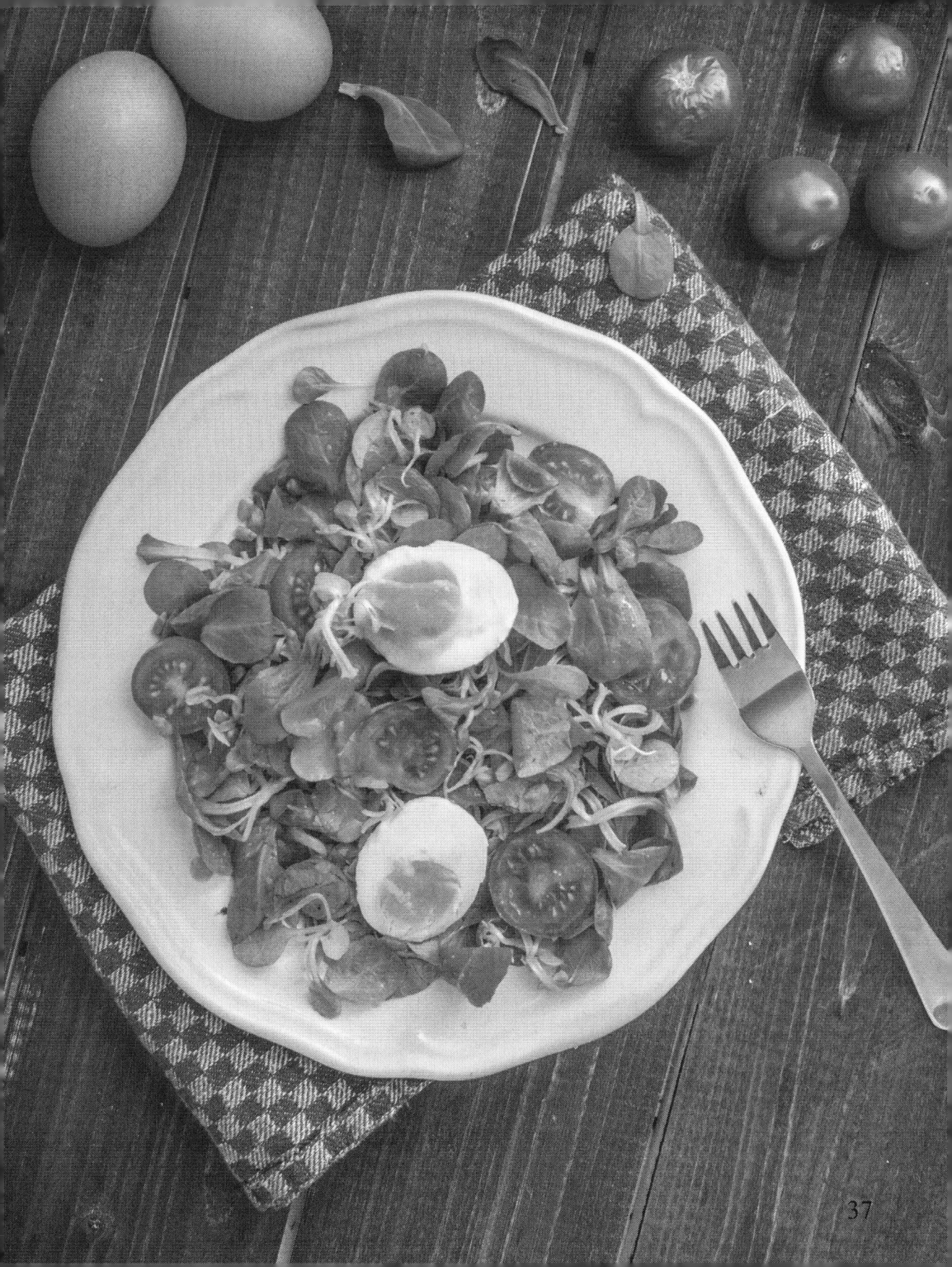

VEGGIE BREAKFAST BOWL

 Cooking Difficulty: 2/10

 Cooking Time: 5 minutes

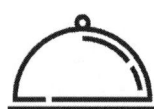 Servings: 1

INGREDIENTS

- 1 egg
- 1 tbsp. water
- 2 tbsps. diced mushrooms
- ¼ c. baby spinach
- 2 tbsps. cherry tomatoes

DESCRIPTION

STEP 1
Mix all ingredients in a greased microwaveable bowl.

STEP 2
Microwave for 1 minute or until the egg is cooked.

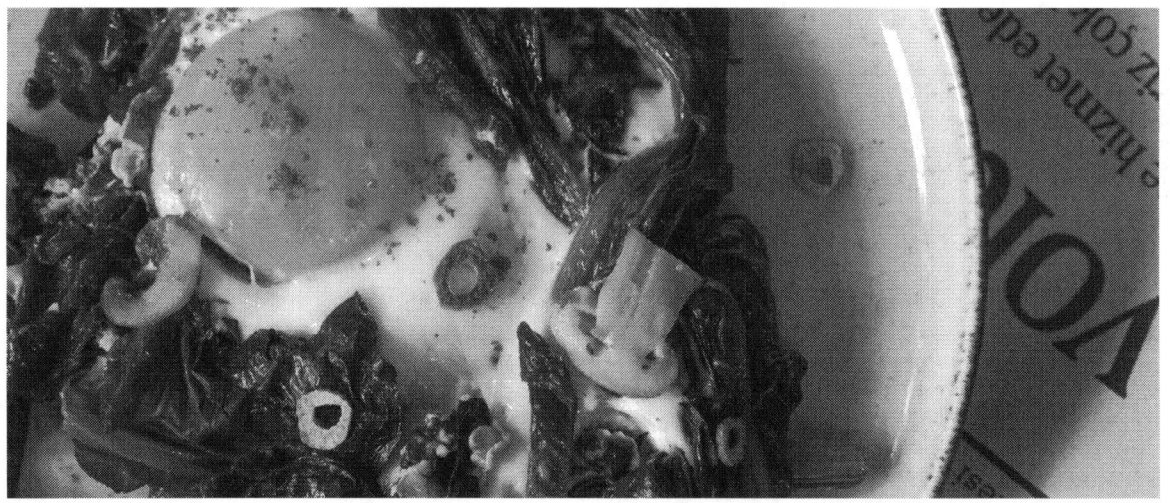

NUTRITIONAL INFORMATION

2g Carbs, 6g Fat, 10g Protein, 100 Calories

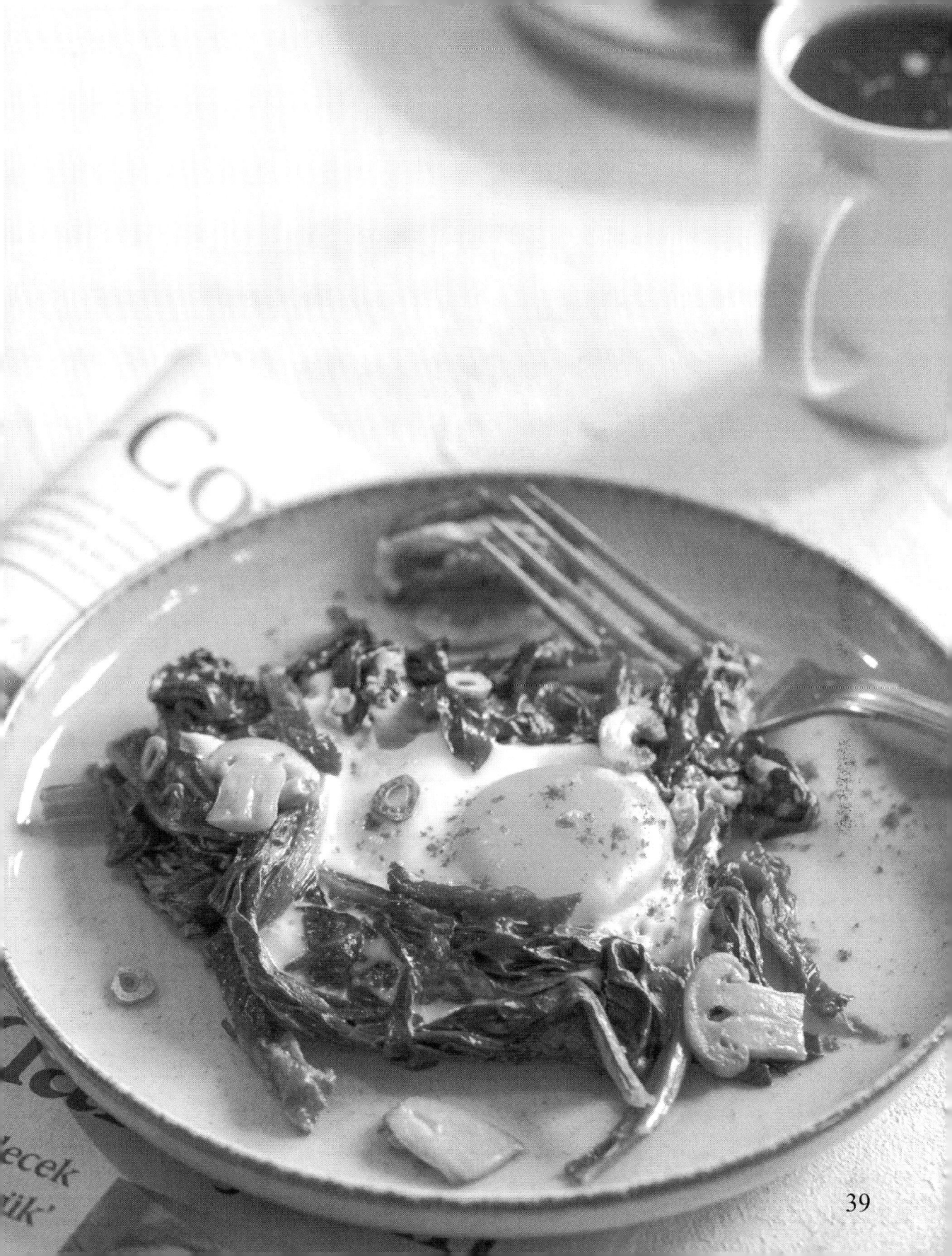

CAJUN TOFU SCRAMBLE

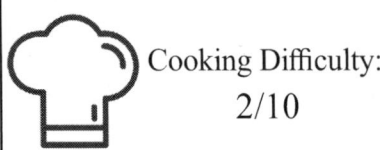 Cooking Difficulty: 2/10

 Cooking Time: 9 minutes

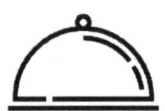 Servings: 2

INGREDIENTS

- 14 ounces drained and cubed tofu
- ½ yellow onion
- 1 diced red bell pepper
- 1 diced zucchini
- 2 teaspoon cajun seasoning
- kale

DESCRIPTION

STEP 1
Saute onions in a skillet until transparent.

STEP 2
Add tofu and seasonings.

STEP 3
Cook for five minutes.

STEP 4
Add vegetables and cook until tender, approximately eight minutes.

NUTRITIONAL INFORMATION

224 Calories, 12g Fats, 11g Net Carbs, 12g Protein

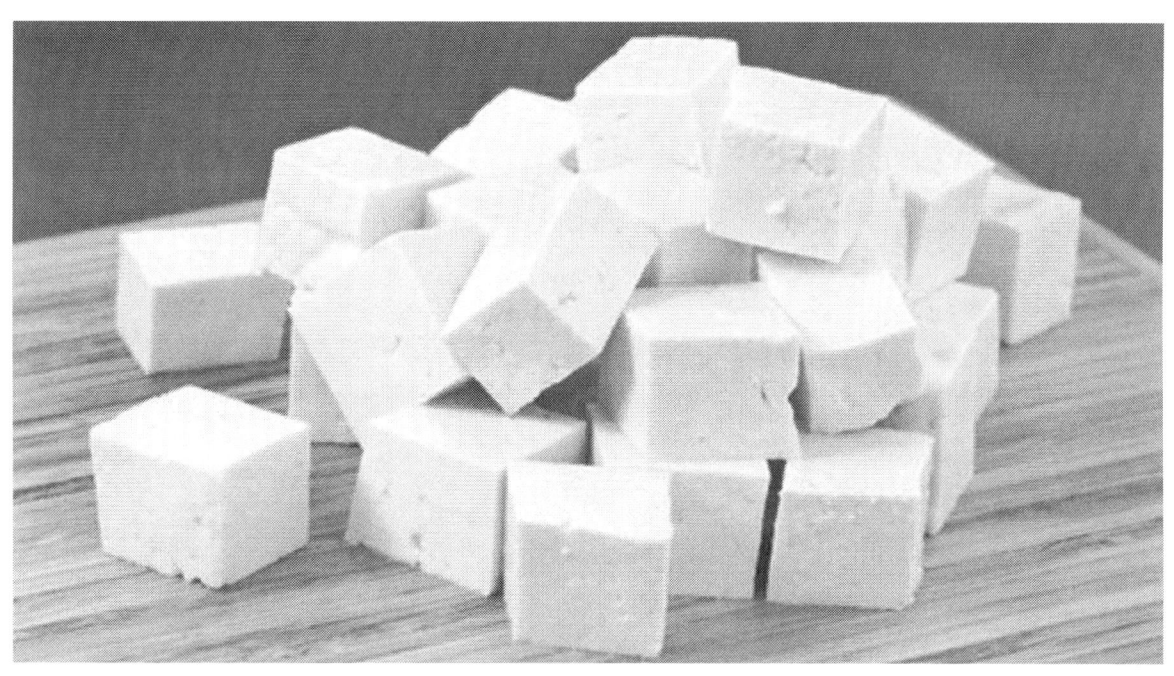

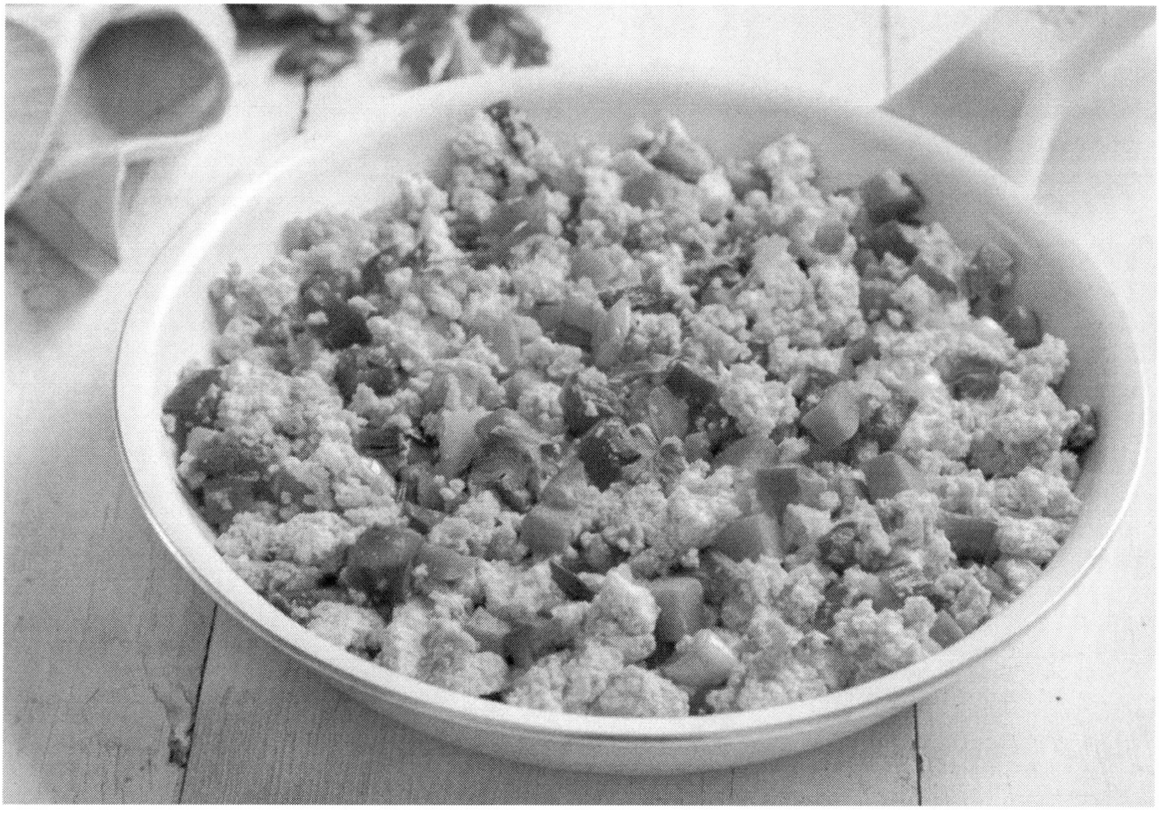

ZUCCHINI PANCAKE WITH GUACAMOLE

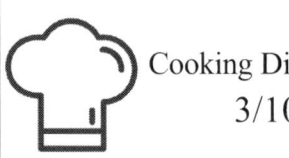 Cooking Difficulty: 3/10	 Cooking Time: 11 minutes	 Servings: 3

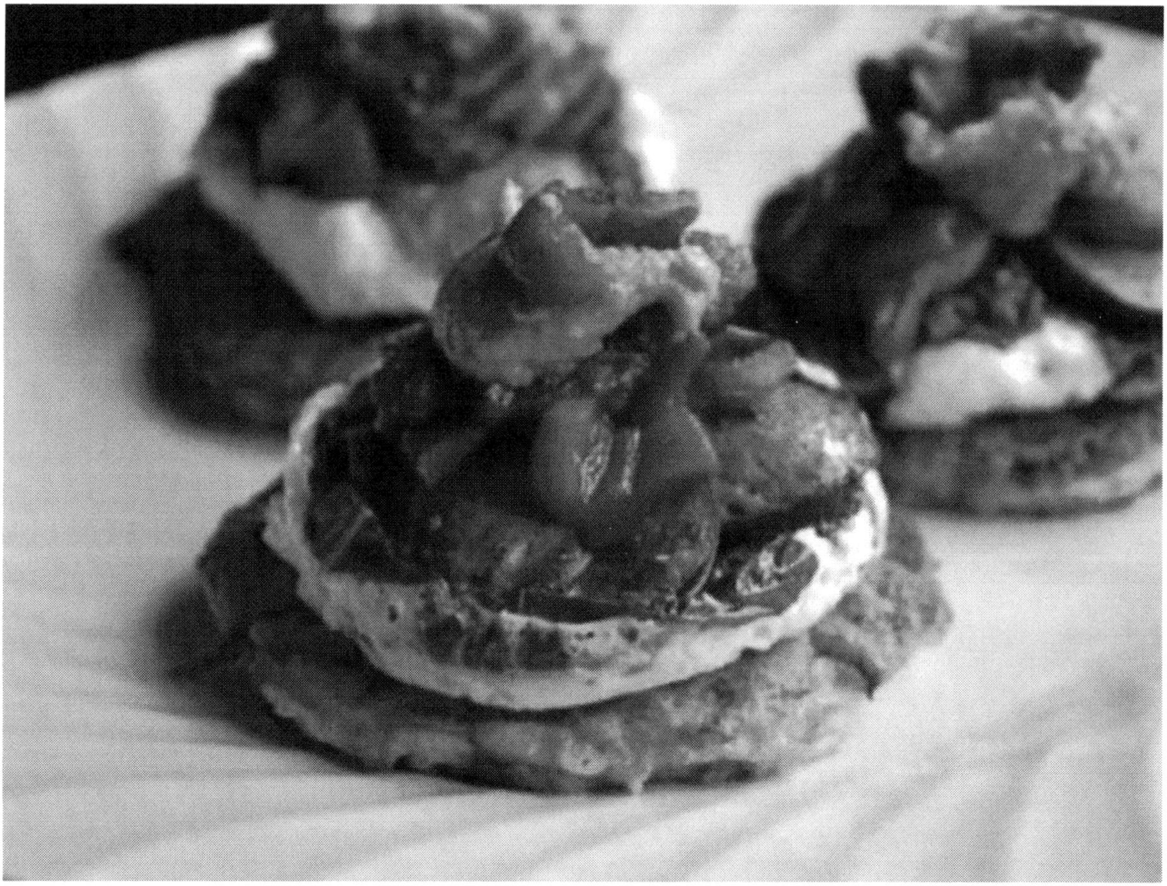

NUTRITIONAL INFORMATION

211 Calories, 14g Fat, 4g Carbs, 4g Protein

INGREDIENTS

for pancake
- 3 egg
- 1 shredded zucchini
- 2 tbsps. coconut flour

for the topping
- 2 large eggs
- ½ c. fresh spinach
- 2 oz. turkey kielbasa
- 3 tbsps. guacamole
- 2 tbsps. jarred roasted red peppers, diced

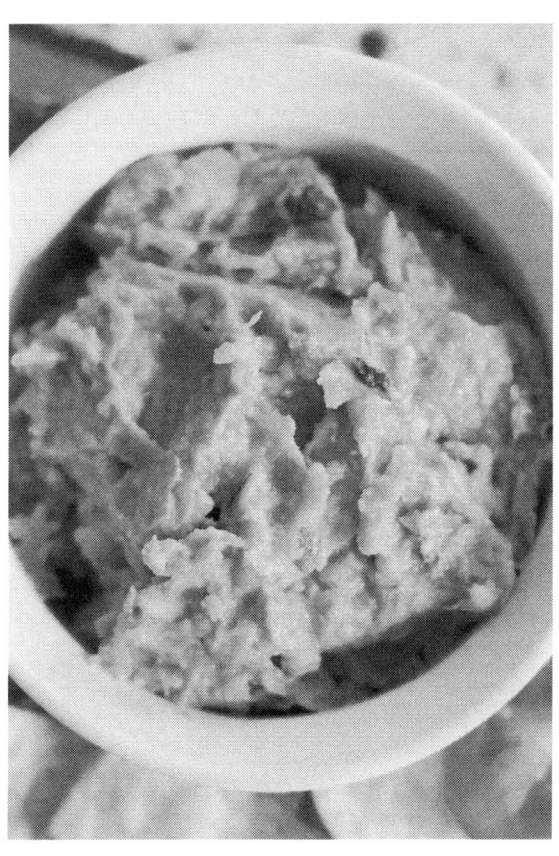

DESCRIPTION

STEP 1
Remove the water in zucchini by squeezing it. Combine the shredded zucchini with flour and egg. Add pepper to taste.

STEP 2
To form the mixture into 3 pancakes, use a non-stick skillet.

STEP 3
Over low heat, cook the mixture for about 3 mins. On each side or until the inside cooks first before the outside burns. Set aside.

STEP 4
Divide the spinach, turkey kielbasa, and raw egg in small bowls or three 4 ounce ramekins. Microwave until you achieve the desired doneness of the eggs or for about 1 minute.

STEP 5
Place egg, kielbasa, spinach layer on top of each pancake, and then add the diced red peppers and guacamole on top.

STRAWBERRY YOGURT

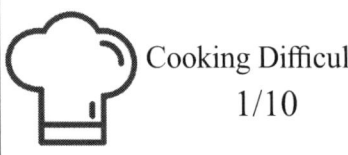 Cooking Difficulty: 1/10	 Cooking Time: 10 minutes	 Servings: 2

INGREDIENTS

- 1 c. strawberry halved
- 2 c. yogurt

DESCRIPTION

STEP 1

In a bowl, combine the yogurt with the strawberry, and toss and keep in the fridge for 10 minutes.

STEP 2

Divide into bowls and serve breakfast.

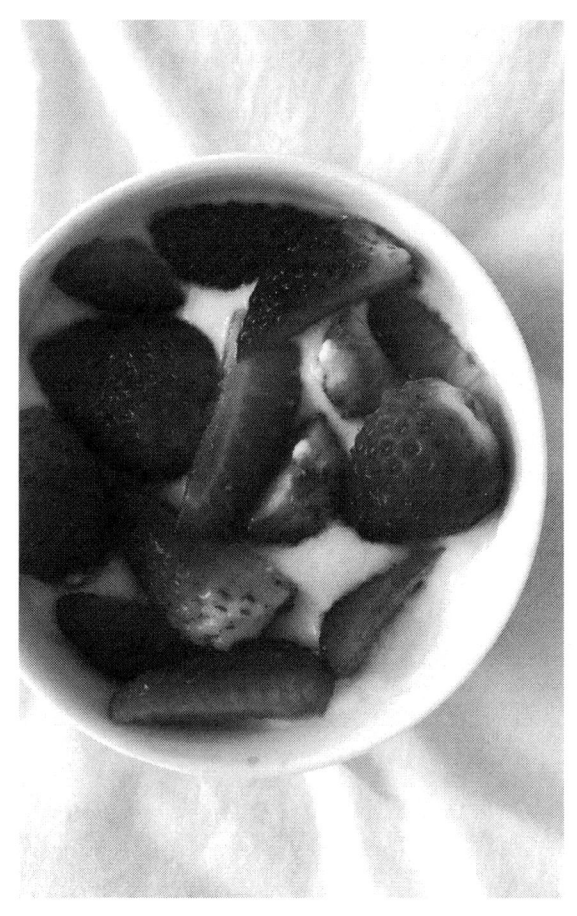

NUTRITIONAL INFORMATION

Calories: 79, Fat: 0.4 g, Carbs: 15 g, Protein: 1.3 g

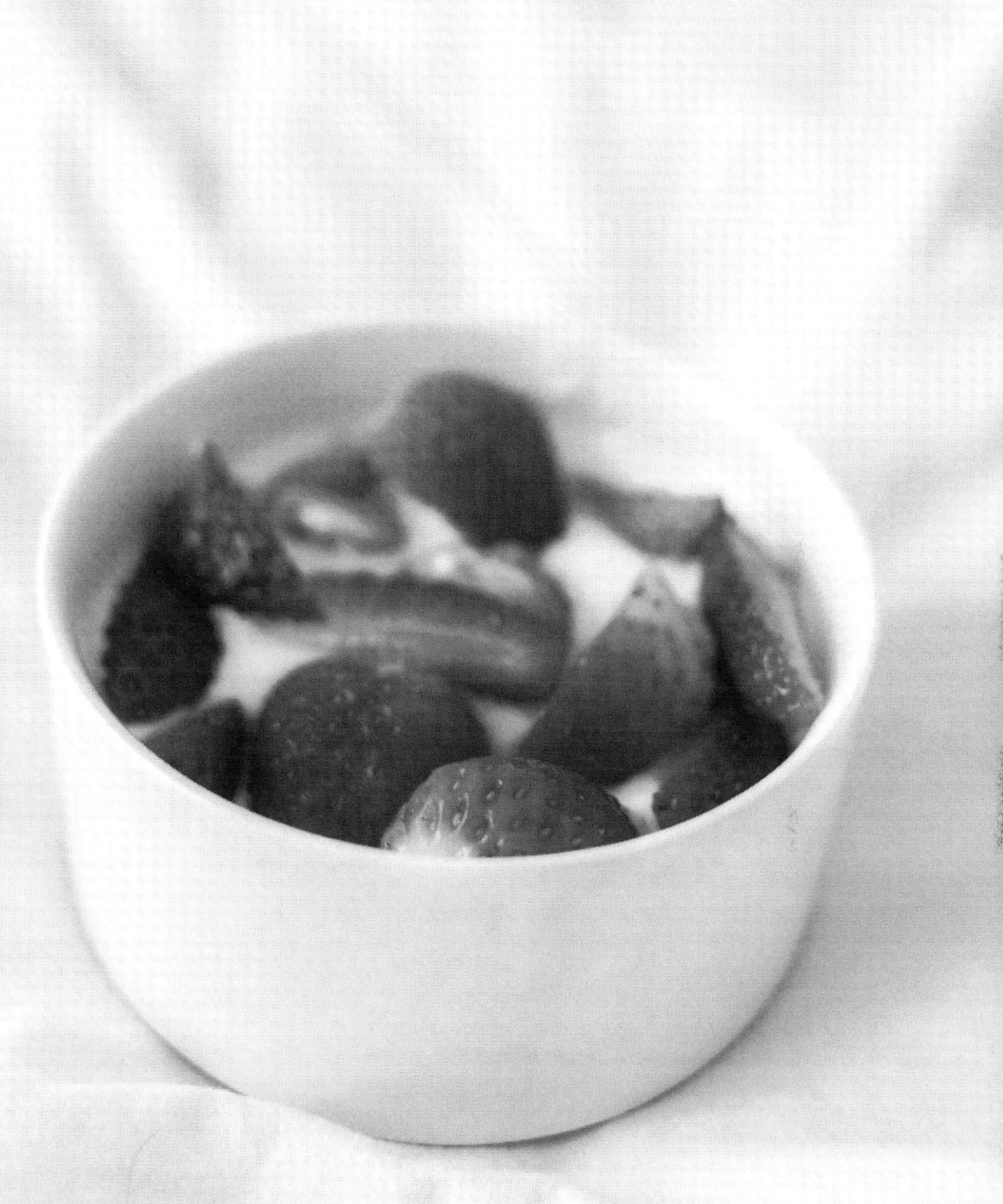

GREEN EGGS

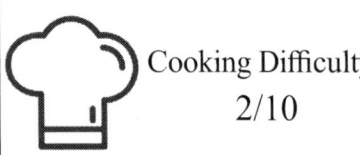 Cooking Difficulty: 2/10

 Cooking Time: 9 minutes

 Servings: 2

INGREDIENTS

- ¼ tsp. ground cayenne
- ¼ tsp. ground cumin
- 4 eggs
- ½ c. chopped parsley
- ½ c. chopped cilantro
- 1 tsp. thyme leaves
- 2 garlic cloves
- 2 tbsp. olive oil

DESCRIPTION

STEP 1
Olive oil in a skillet before adding the garlic and frying.

STEP 2
Add in the thyme, parsley, and cilantro and cook another 3 minutes.

STEP 3
At this time, add in the eggs and season. Cover with a lid and let this cook for another 5 minutes before serving.

NUTRITIONAL INFORMATION

211 Calories, 7g Fats, 4g Carbs, 12.8 Protein

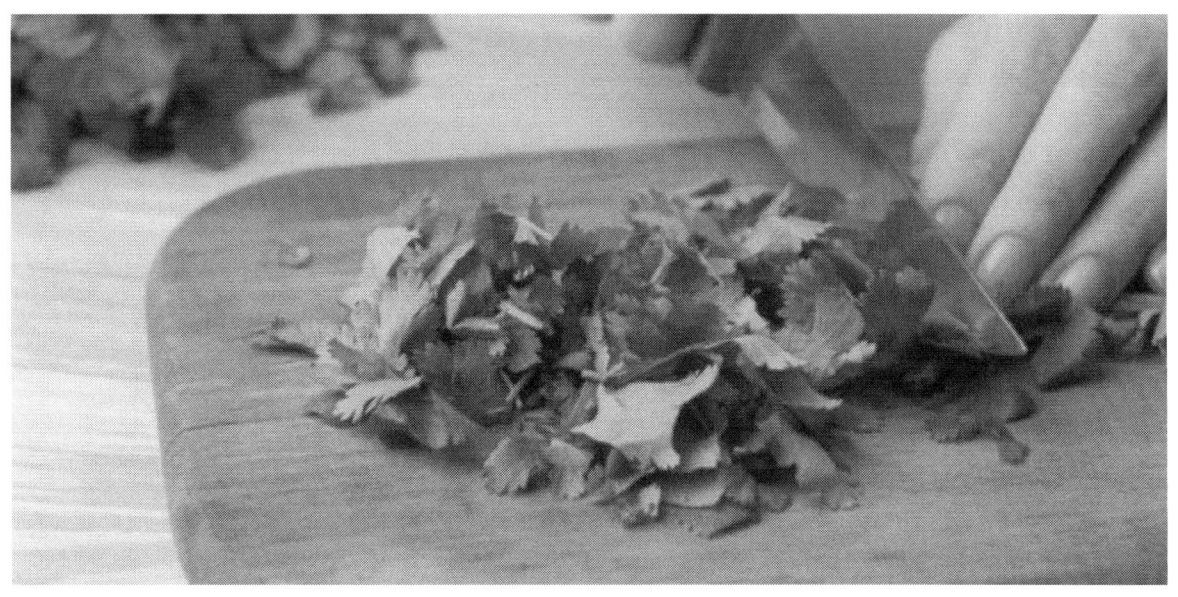

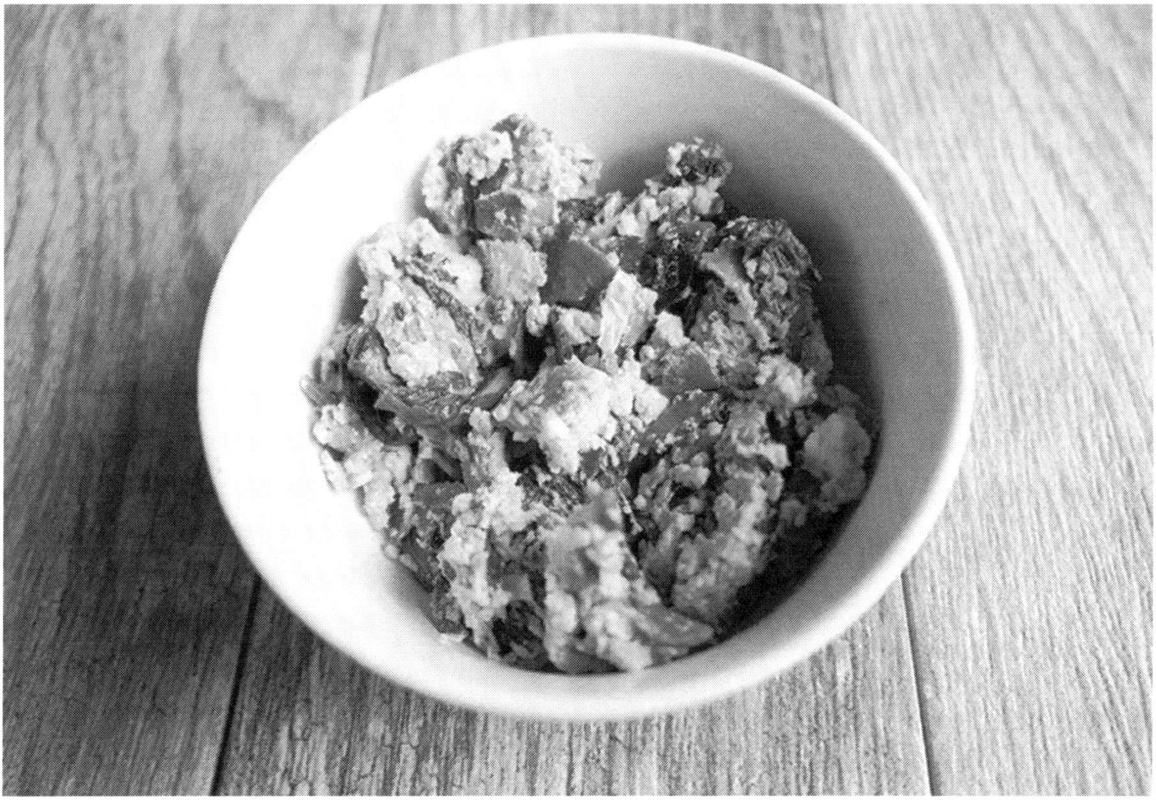

CHIA SEED PUDDING

 Cooking Difficulty: 1/10  Cooking Time: 12 minutes 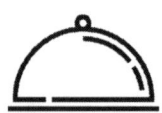 Servings: 1

INGREDIENTS

- 1/2 cup coconut milk
- 2 tbsp. chia seeds
- berries

DESCRIPTION

STEP 1
Combine chia seeds and milk in a large bowl. Let the mixture sit for 10 minutes, then stir again as soon as the chia seeds begin to swell.

STEP 2
Cover the bowl with a lid and refrigerate for an hour or more.

STEP 3
Stir the chia pudding before serving and add your favorite berries. Enjoy!

NUTRITIONAL INFORMATION

180 Calories, 3 g Fat, 3g Carbs, 3g Protein

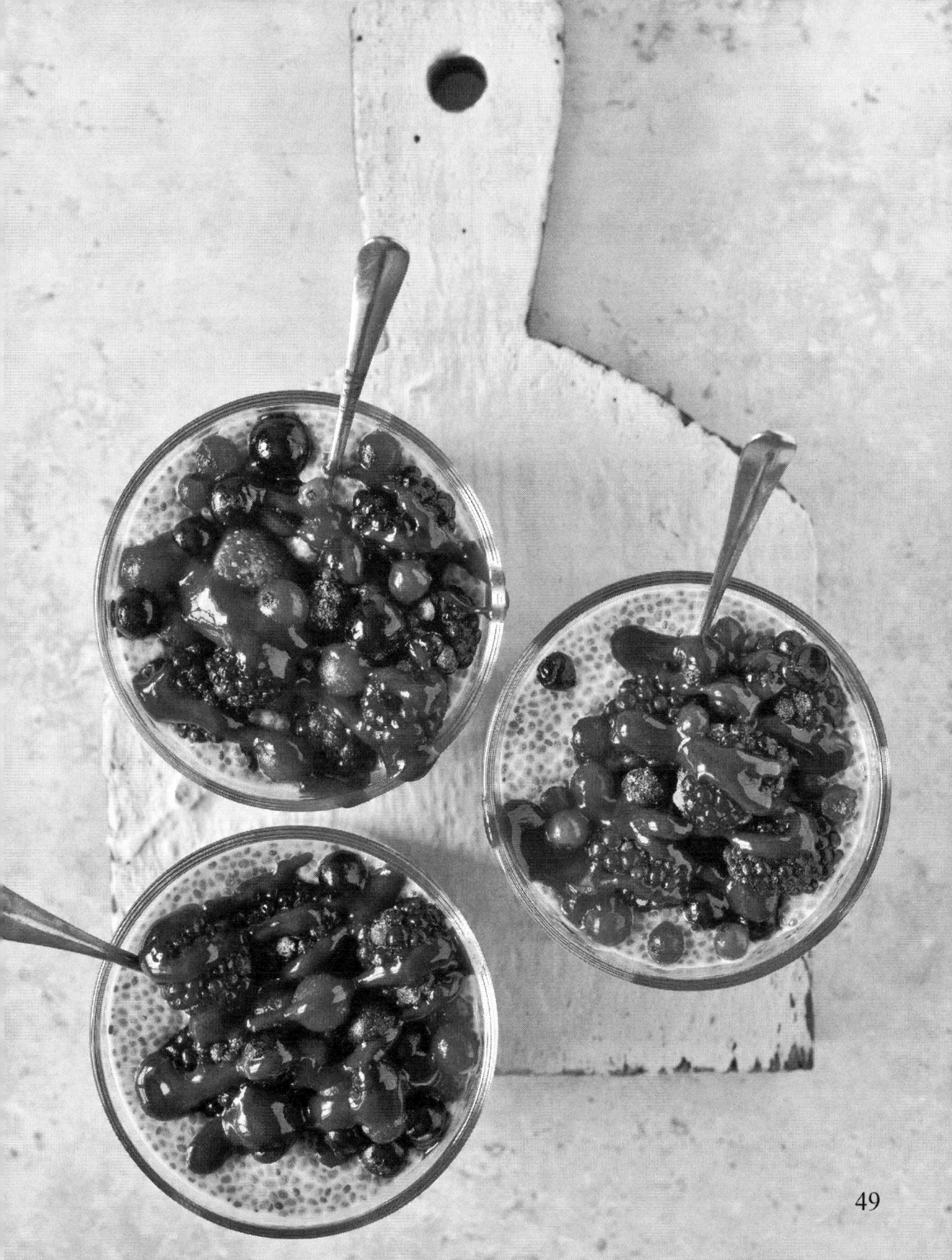

EDAMAME & SWEET PEA HUMMUS

 Cooking Difficulty: 1/10

 Cooking Time: 5 minutes

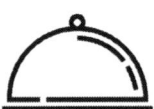 Servings: 2

INGREDIENTS

- ½ c. edamame
- ½ c. peas
- 2 tbsps. tahini
- 1 minced garlic clove
- 2 tbsps. chopped mint
- 3 tbsps. olive oil
- 2 wheat tortillas
- 2 eggs

DESCRIPTION

STEP 1
Blend the first 5 ingredients and 1 Tbsp. Of olive oil in a food processor. Spread evenly over the wheat tortillas.

STEP 2
Coat the pan with the remaining olive oil and cook the eggs. When ready, put one egg on each tortilla.

NUTRITIONAL INFORMATION

15g Carbs, 20g Fat, 10g Protein, 260 Calories

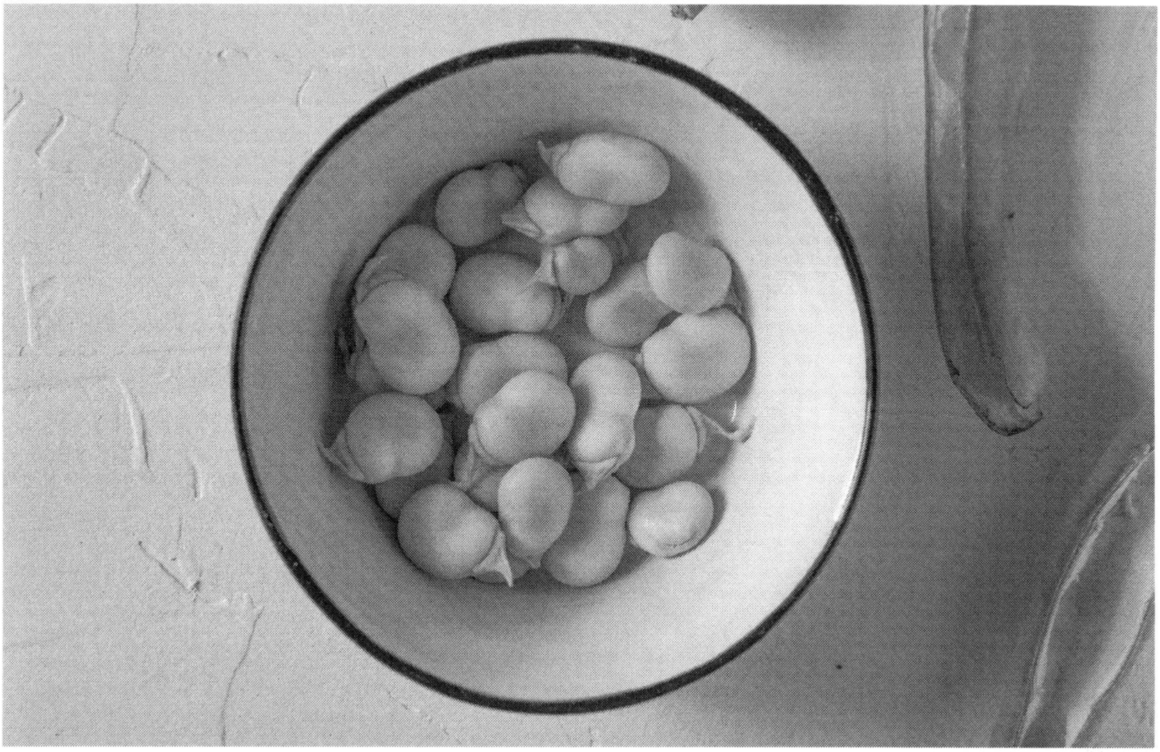

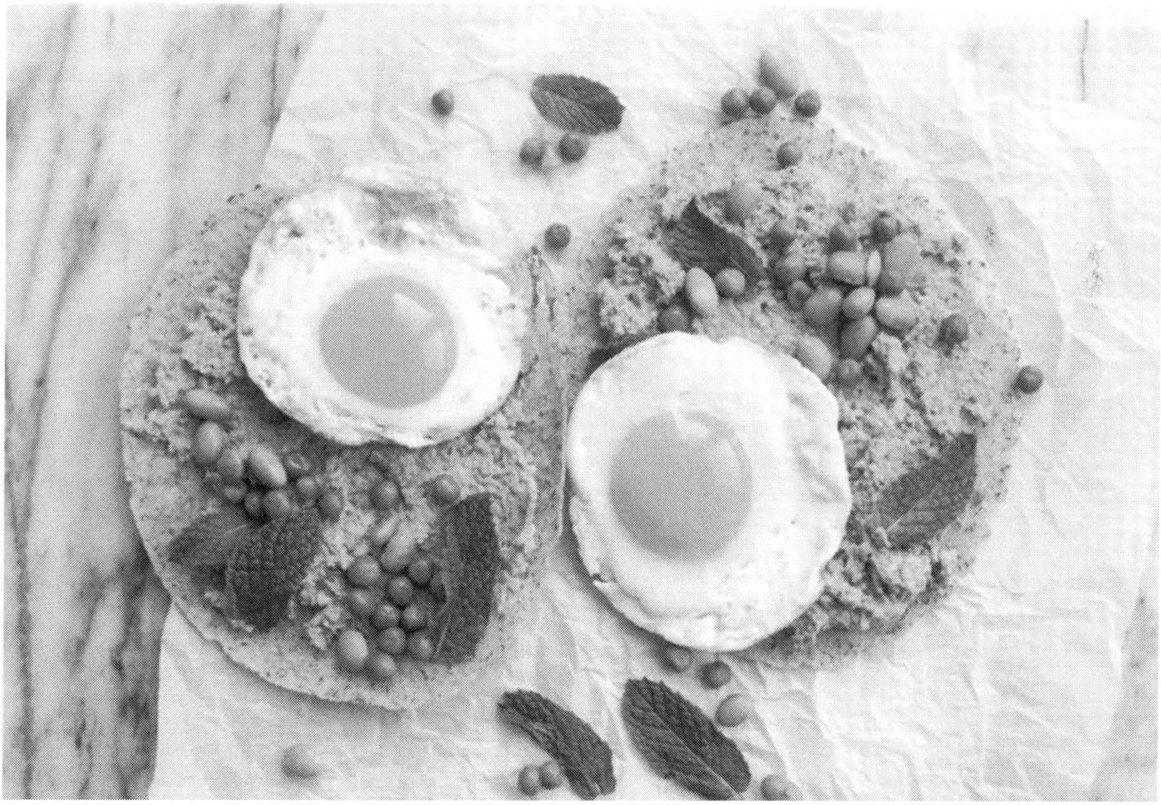

TOMATOES AND EGGS

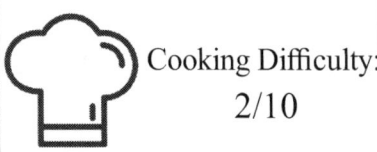 Cooking Difficulty: 2/10

 Cooking Time: 15 minutes

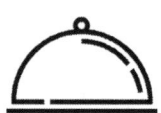 Servings: 2

INGREDIENTS

- 1 tbsp. olive oil
- salt
- black pepper
- dried basil
- 1 tbsp. chopped parsley
- 4 eggs
- 6 tomatoes diced

DESCRIPTION

STEP 1
Heat olive oil in a pan.

STEP 2
Add tomatoes, spices, and herbs. Simmer, stirring, for about 5-7 minutes.

STEP 3
Make small wells in the sauce and break the eggs into them. Season with salt and cook until the white is white and the yolk inside is still runny.

STEP 4
Remove from fire. Sprinkle with parsley before serving.

NUTRITIONAL INFORMATION

Calories: 310, Fat: 4 g, Carbs: 5 g, Protein: 3 g

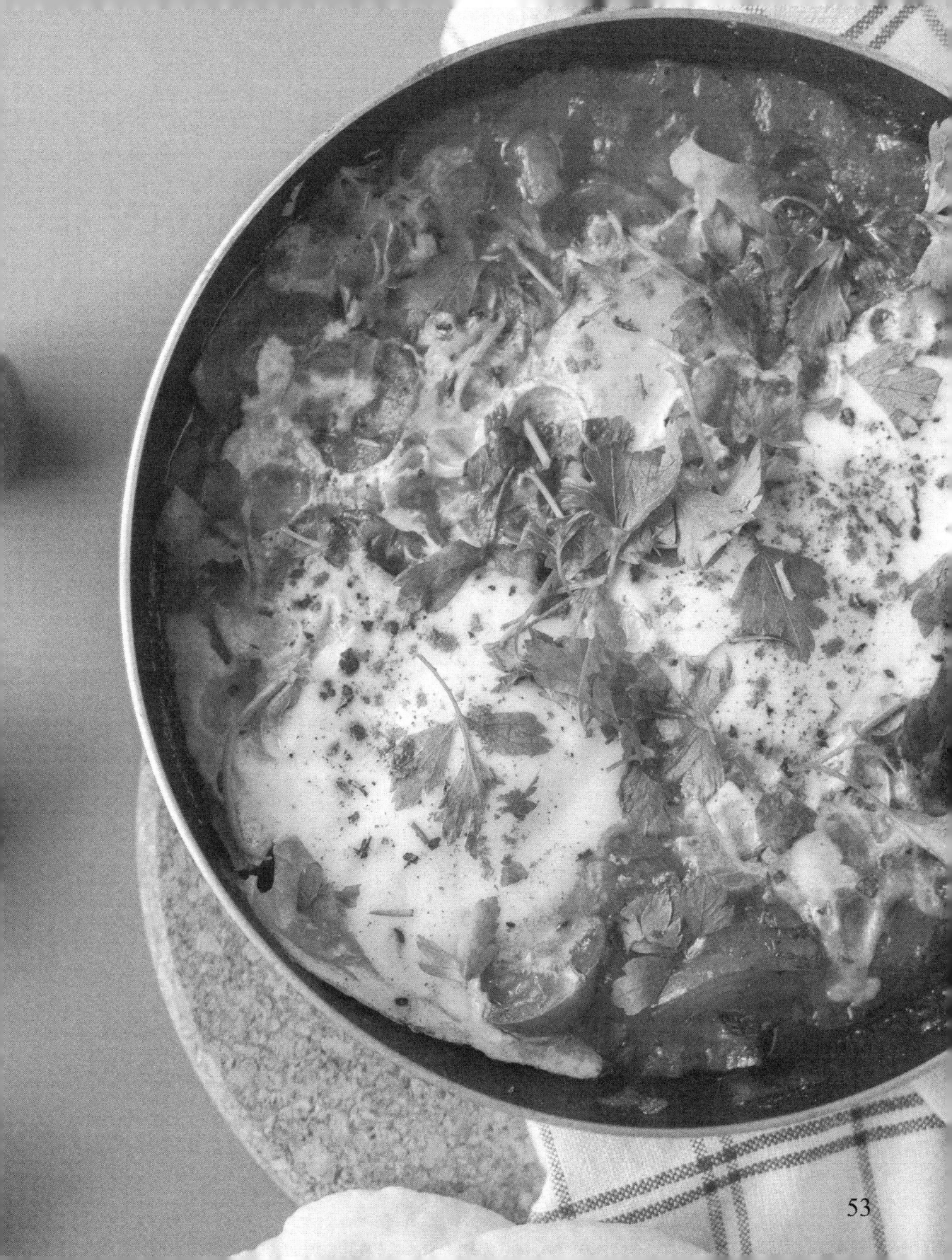

TOFU SCRAMBLE TOAST

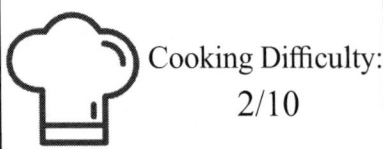 Cooking Difficulty:
2/10

 Cooking Time:
7 minutes

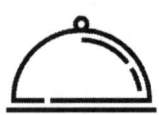 Servings:
2

INGREDIENTS

- 14 ounces of drained and diced tofu
- ½ yellow onion
- 2 teaspoons cajun seasoning
- 2 toasted bread
- favorite vegetables for serving

DESCRIPTION

STEP 1
Heat a frying pan and add a little olive oil.

STEP 2
Add tofu and spices. Cook for 5 minutes.

STEP 3
Fry one side of the toast. Place tofu on toast. Garnish with your favorite vegetables. Serve for breakfast.

NUTRITIONAL INFORMATION

247 Calories, 5.8g Fats, 6g Carbs, 10g Protein

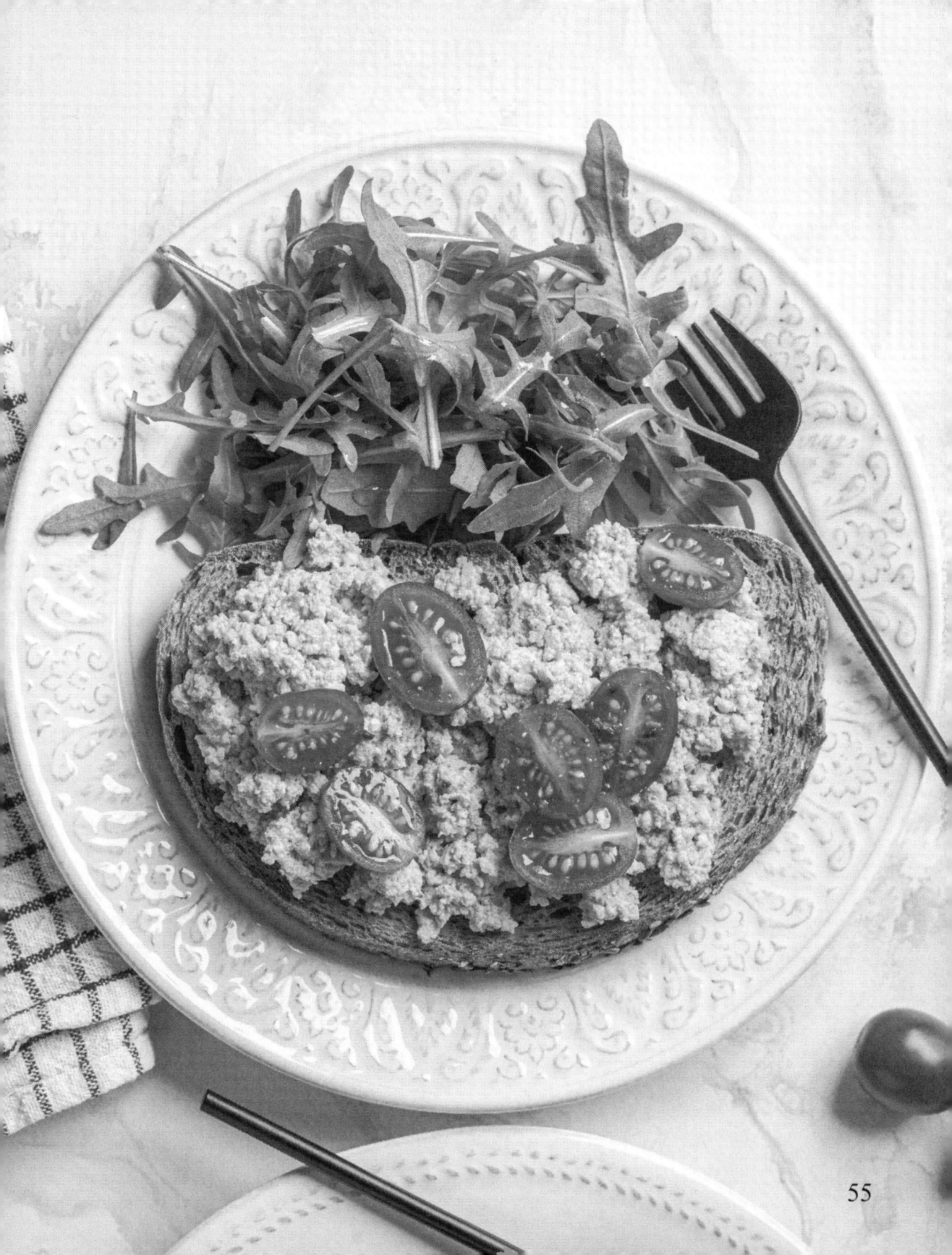

AVOCADO SPREAD

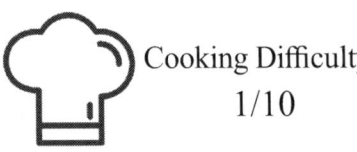 Cooking Difficulty: 1/10

 Cooking Time: 1 minutes

 Servings: 4

INGREDIENTS

- 3 peeled and pitted avocados, chopped
- 1 tbsp. olive oil
- 1 tbsp. lime juice
- salt
- black pepper
- 1 tbsp. chopped chives
- 4 eggs
- wholemeal bread

DESCRIPTION

STEP 1
In a blender, mix the avocado pulp with oil and other ingredients.

STEP 2
Heat a skillet over low heat and add olive oil. Fry eggs until done.

STEP 3
Spread guacamole on bread and top with a fried egg.

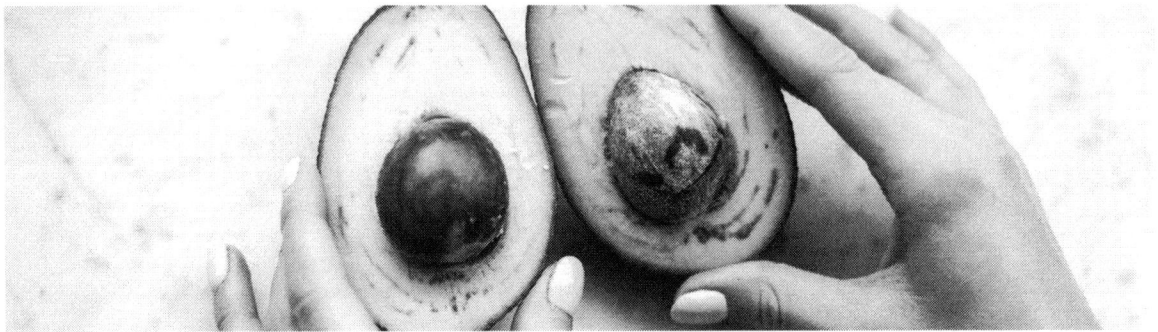

NUTRITIONAL INFORMATION

Calories: 79, Fat: 0.4 g, Carbs: 15 g, Protein: 1.3 g

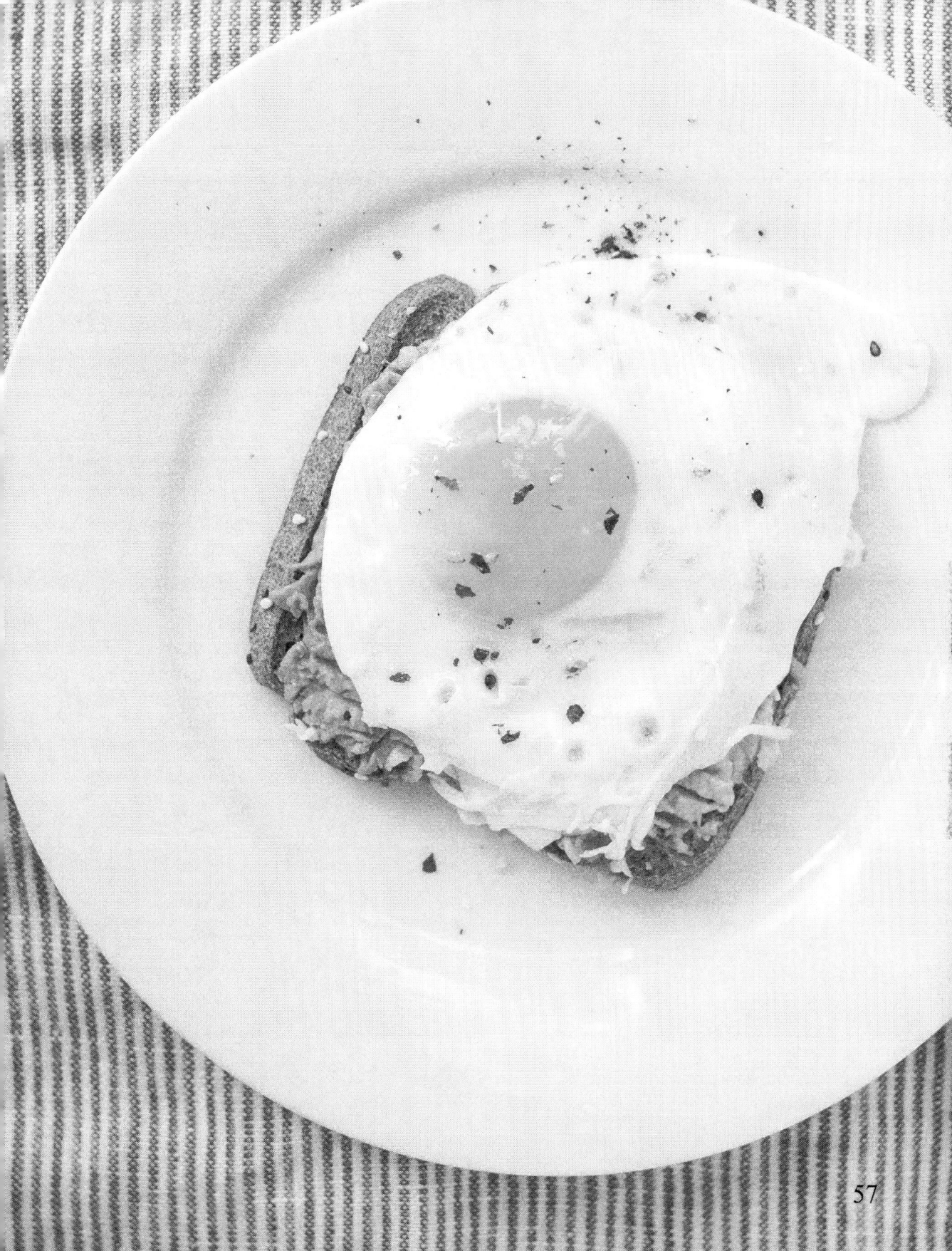

GRANOLA WITH GRAPEFRUIT

 Cooking Difficulty: 1/10

 Cooking Time: 3 minutes

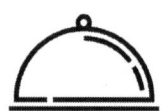 Servings: 2

INGREDIENTS

- 1/2 cup coconut cream
- 6 tbsp. granola
- grapefruit

DESCRIPTION

STEP 1
Take two cups. Place 3 spoonfuls of granola in each one.

STEP 2
Then place the coconut cream on top of the granola.

STEP 3
Garnish everything with grapefruit. Enjoy your meal.

NUTRITIONAL INFORMATION

111 Calories, 6g Fats, 3g Carbs, 6.8 Protein

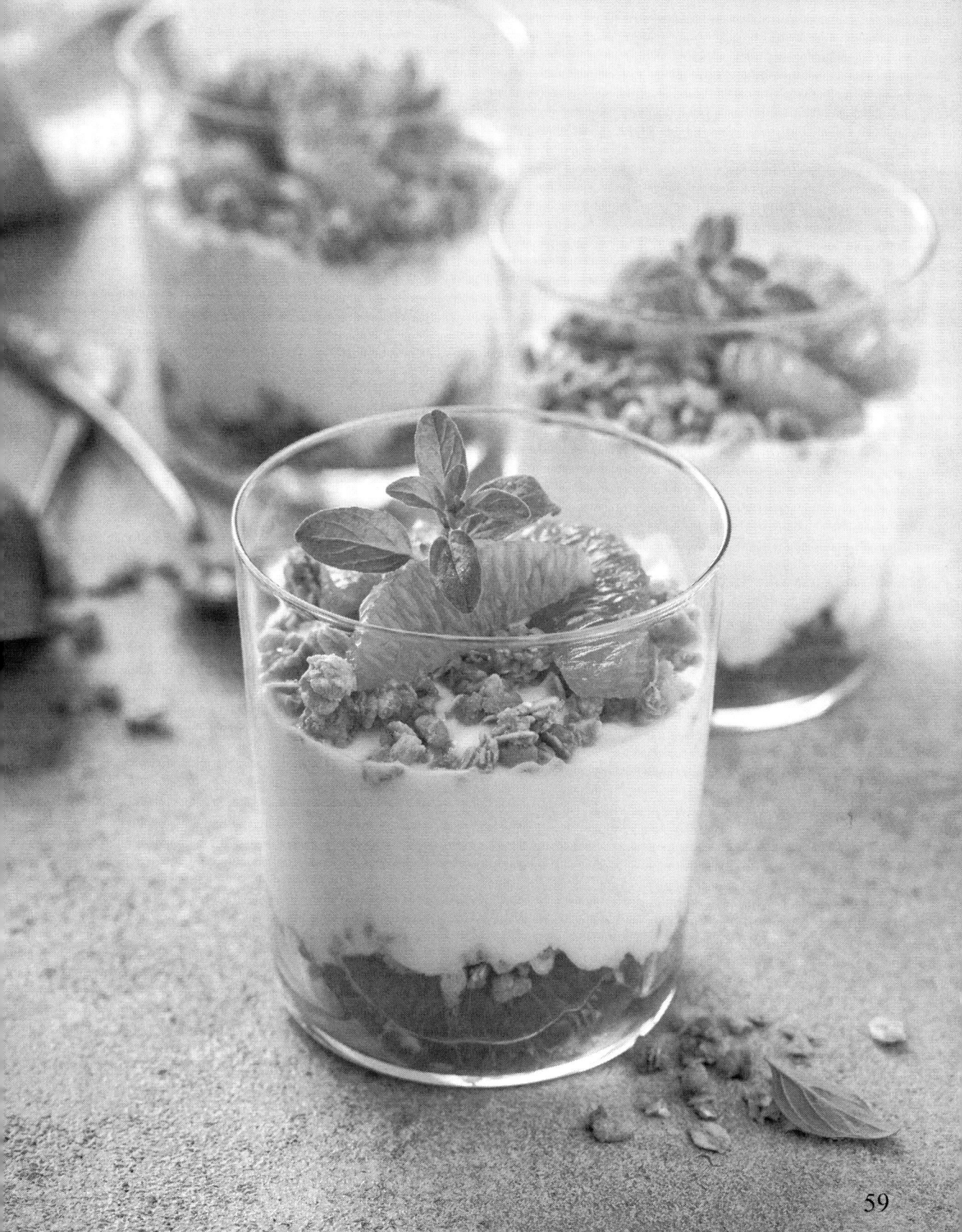

SPINACH SMOOTHIE

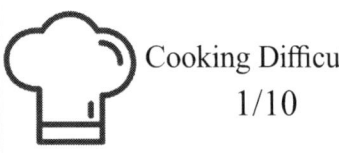 Cooking Difficulty: 1/10	 Cooking Time: 1 minutes	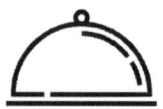 Servings: 1

INGREDIENTS

- 3c. spinach
- 1 c. chopped kale leaves
- 2 c. water
- mint leaves
- ice cubes

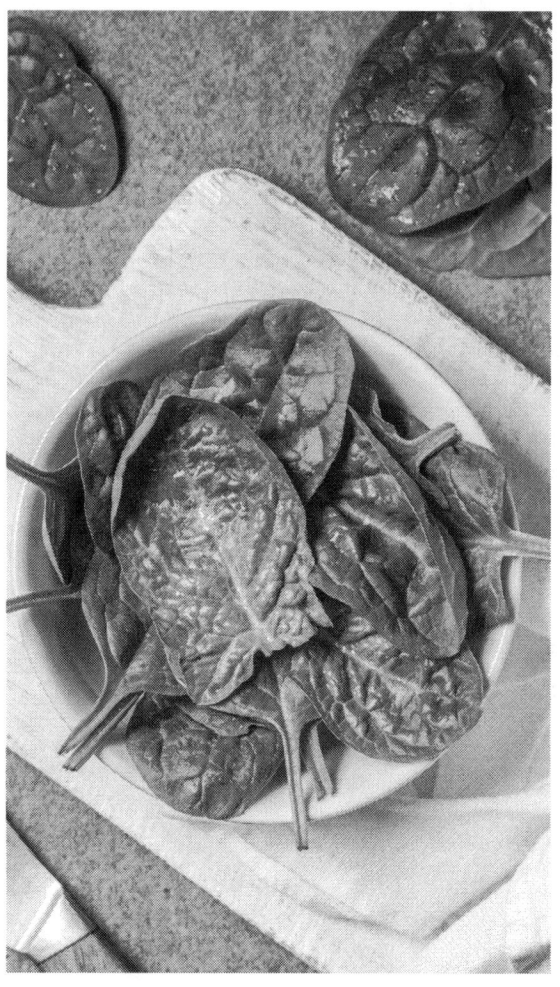

DESCRIPTION

STEP 1
Except for the mint leaves, add everything in a blender and blend until smooth.

STEP 2
Garnish with mint leaves and serve.

NUTRITIONAL INFORMATION

Calories: 79, Fat: 1g, Carbs: 4.9g, Protein: 5g

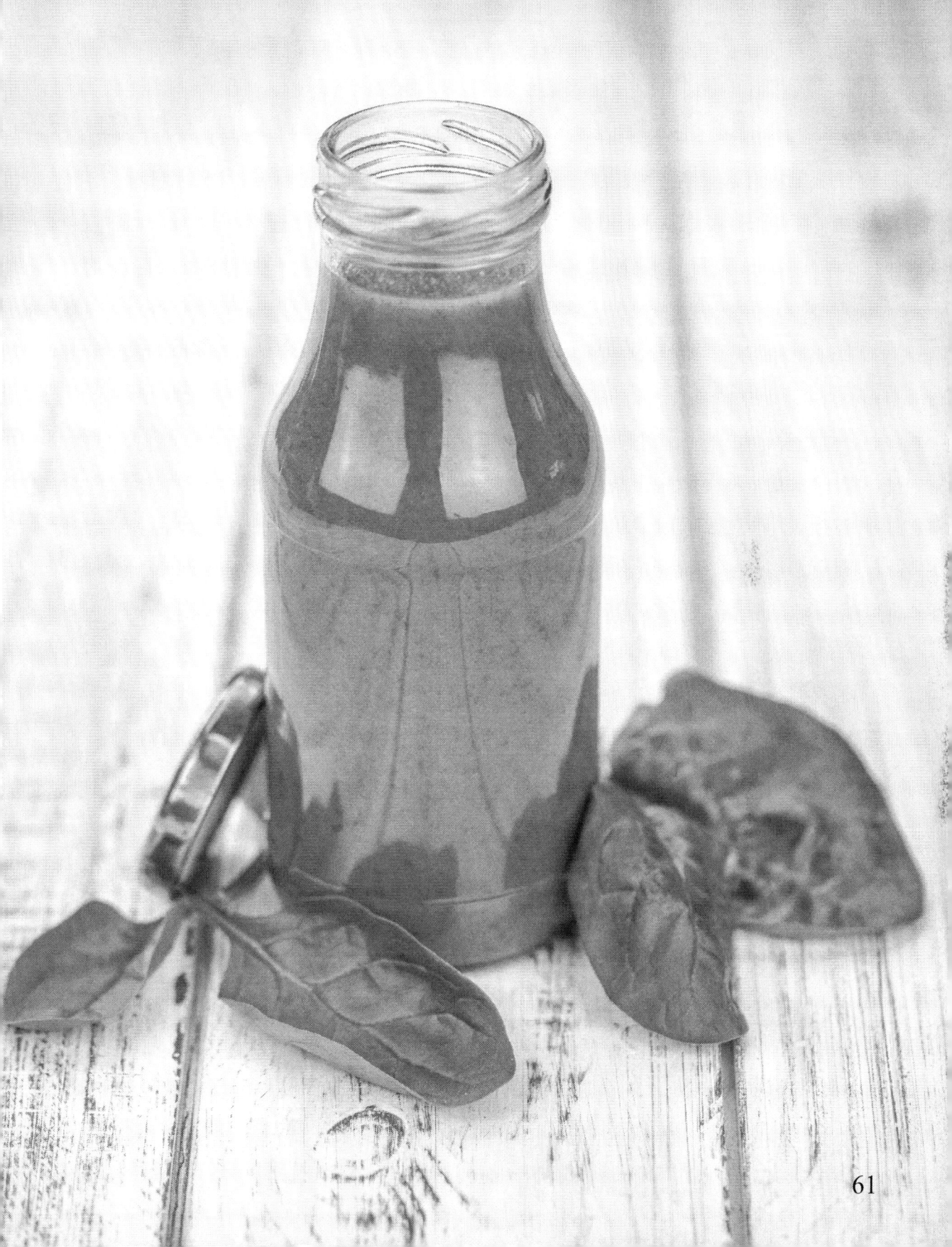

CHILI SPINACH MIX

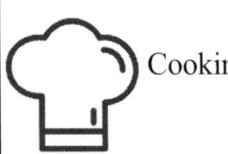 Cooking Difficulty: 3/10

 Cooking Time: 24 minutes

 Servings: 4

INGREDIENTS

- 1 lb. ground chicken meat
- 1 tbsp. avocado oil
- 2 chopped shallots
- 2 minced garlic cloves
- 2 tsps. red chili flakes (optional)
- 1 tbsp. tomato passata
- 1 c. baby spinach
- 1 tsp. chili powder
- salt
- black pepper

DESCRIPTION

STEP 1
Ensure that you heat the pan, add the shallots and the garlic, stir, then cook for 3 minutes.

STEP 2
Add the meat and brown it for 5 minutes.

STEP 3
Add the chili flakes and the other ingredients, toss, cook over medium heat for 15 minutes, divide into bowls and serve for breakfast.

NUTRITIONAL INFORMATION

Calories 239, Fat 9.2g, Carbs 3.2g, Protein 4.1g

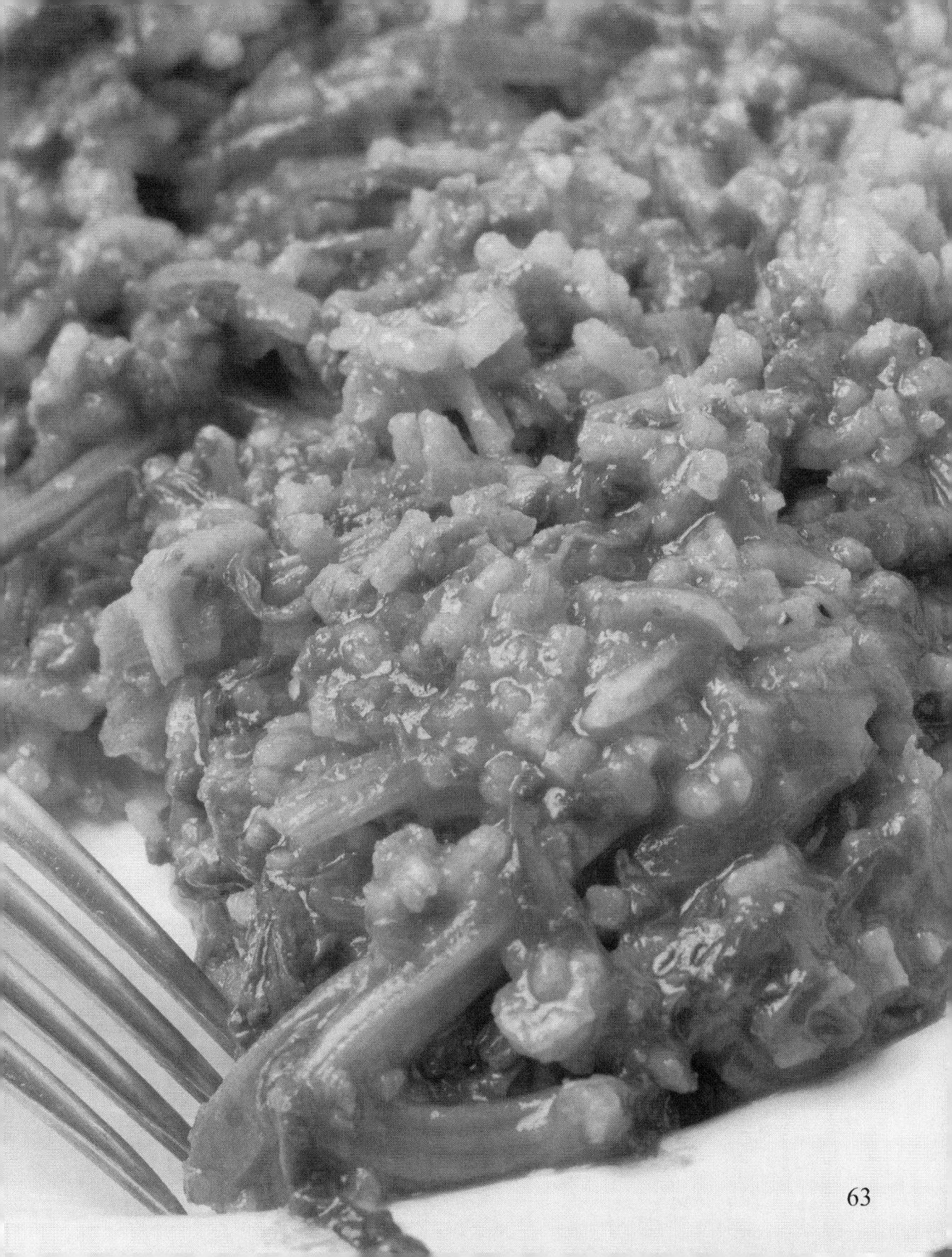

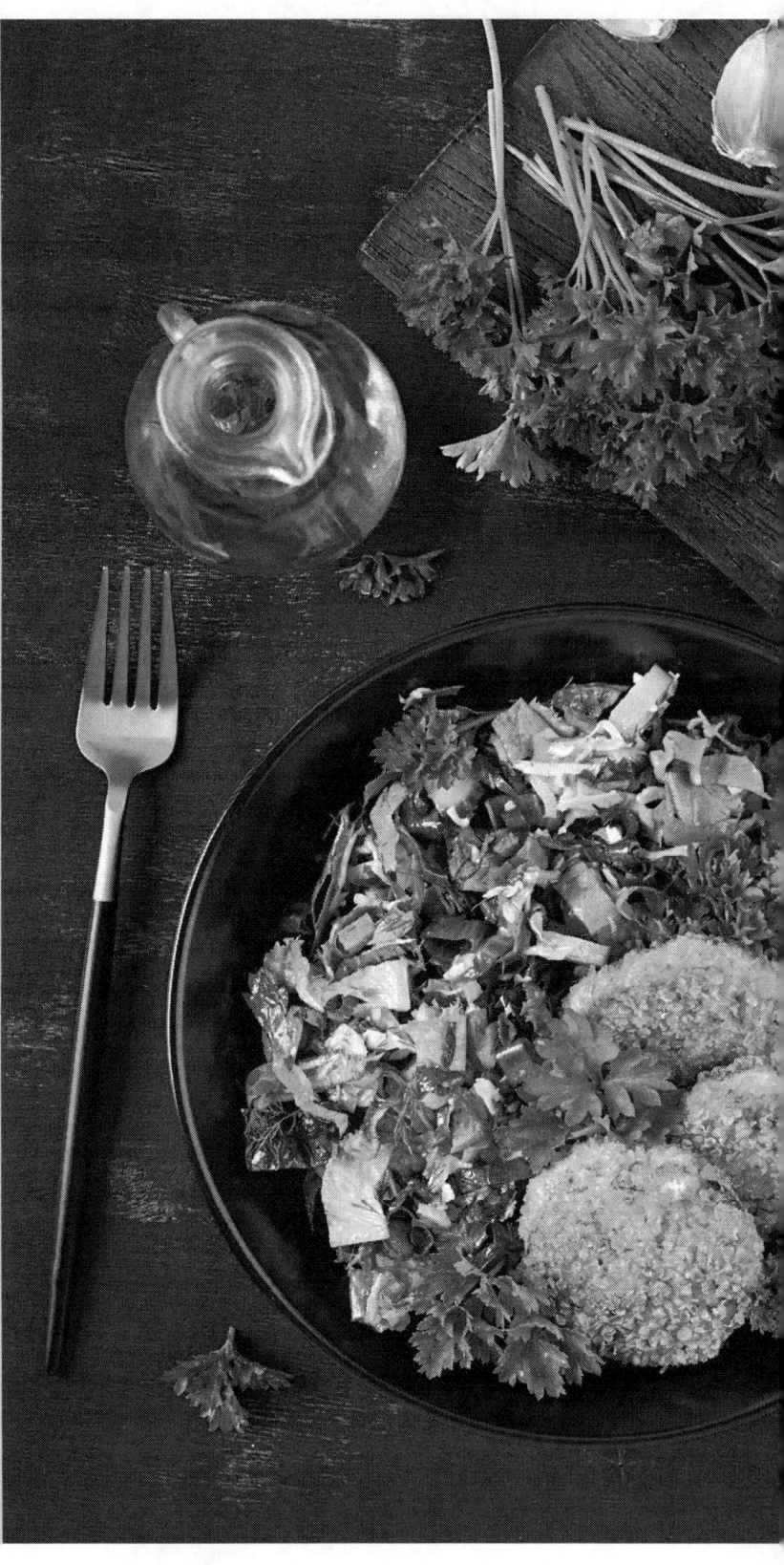

LUNCH RECIPES

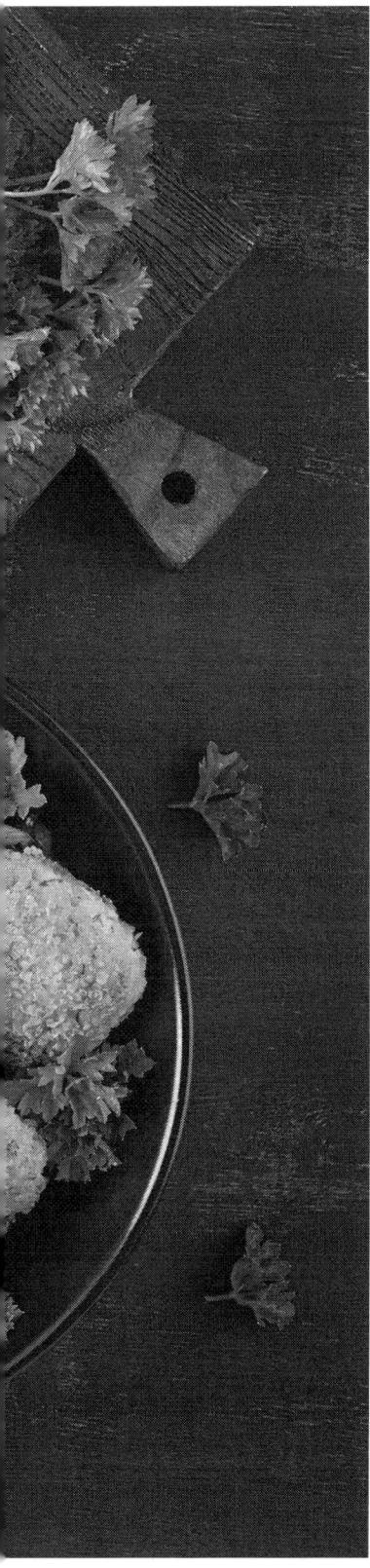

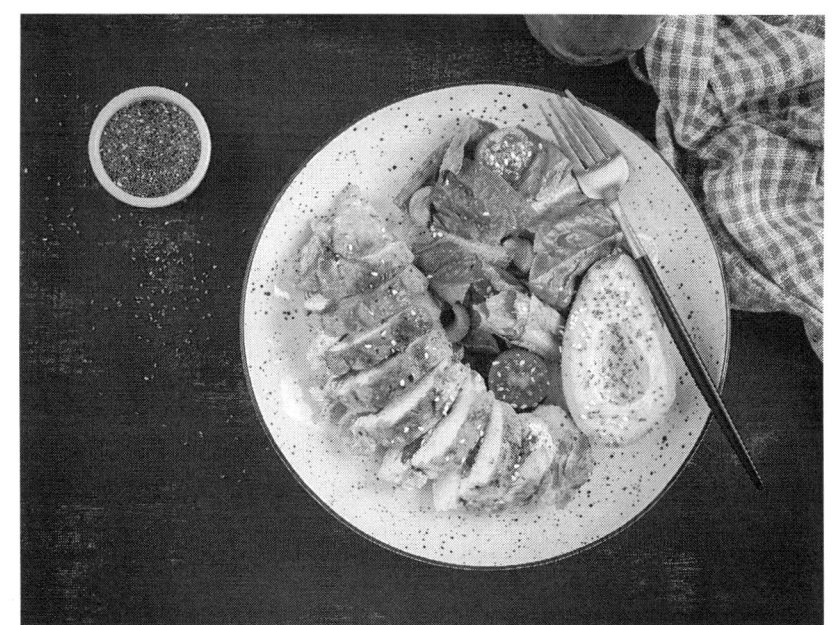

Recipes include foods recommended in the GOLO diet, such as lean sources of protein, lean dairy products, low glycemic index vegetables, whole grains, and healthy sources of fat. Recipes include low to medium GI ingredients to help maintain stable blood sugar levels.

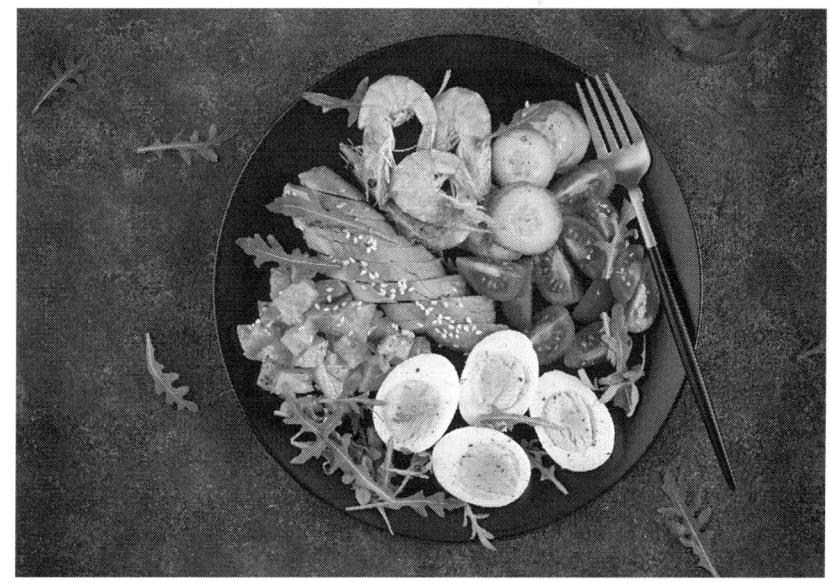

VEGETABLE WRAPS

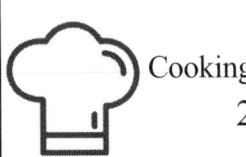 Cooking Difficulty: 2/10

 Cooking Time: 9 minutes

 Servings: 4

INGREDIENTS

- 1 head of romaine lettuce
- 2 carrots
- 1 cucumber
- 1 red onion
- 1 celery stalk
- dressing of choice

DESCRIPTION

STEP 1
Finely slice the carrots, cucumber, red onion, and celery into sticks of vegetable.

STEP 2
Divide between 12 lettuce leaves.

STEP 3
Roll up lettuce leaves and serve.

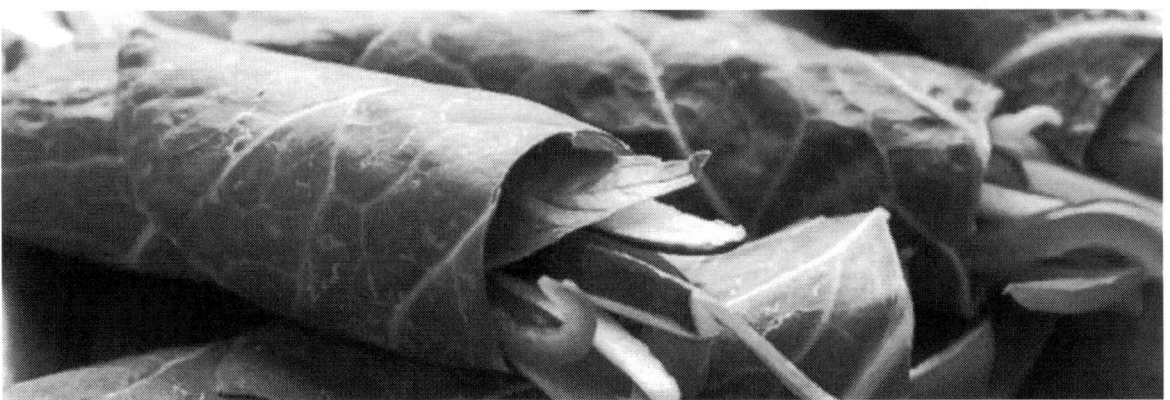

NUTRITIONAL INFORMATION

20 Calories, 6g Fats, 1g Carbs, and 0g Protein

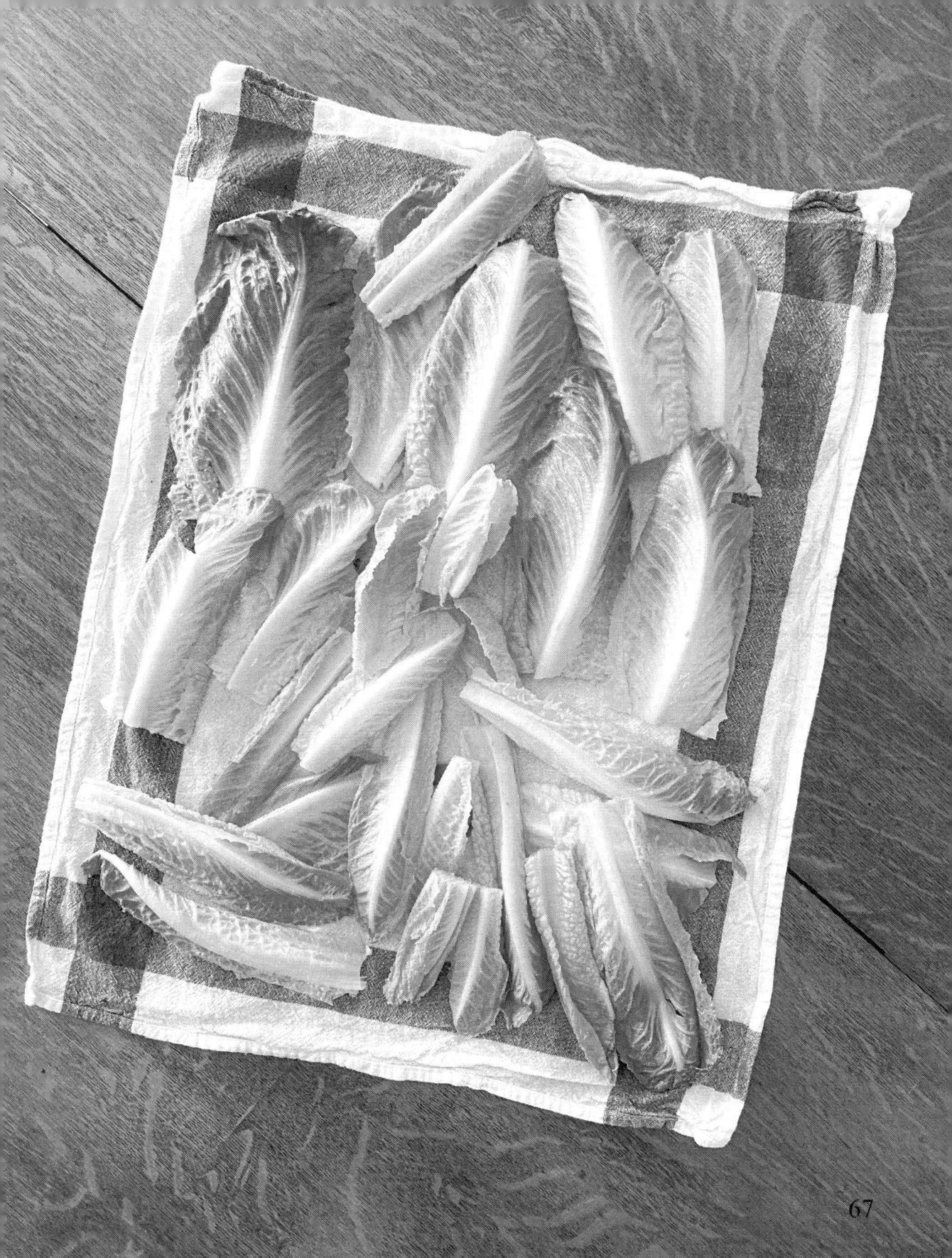

MUSHROOM SOUP

 Cooking Difficulty: 2/10	 Cooking Time: 20 minutes	 Servings: 2

INGREDIENTS

- 1 pound champignons
- 3 shallots
- 2 cloves of garlic
- 2 cups chicken broth
- 7 tbsp. natural yogurt
- 2 tbsp. olive oil

DESCRIPTION

STEP 1
Sauté the finely chopped onion in a saucepan in olive oil until tender.

STEP 2
Add mushrooms and garlic. Then pour chicken broth into a saucepan, bring to a boil and cook for another 10 minutes, until mushrooms are tender.

STEP 3
Whisk the soup with a blender and season with natural yogurt before serving.

NUTRITIONAL INFORMATION

201 Calories, 8.1g Fats, 3g Carbs, 3 Protein

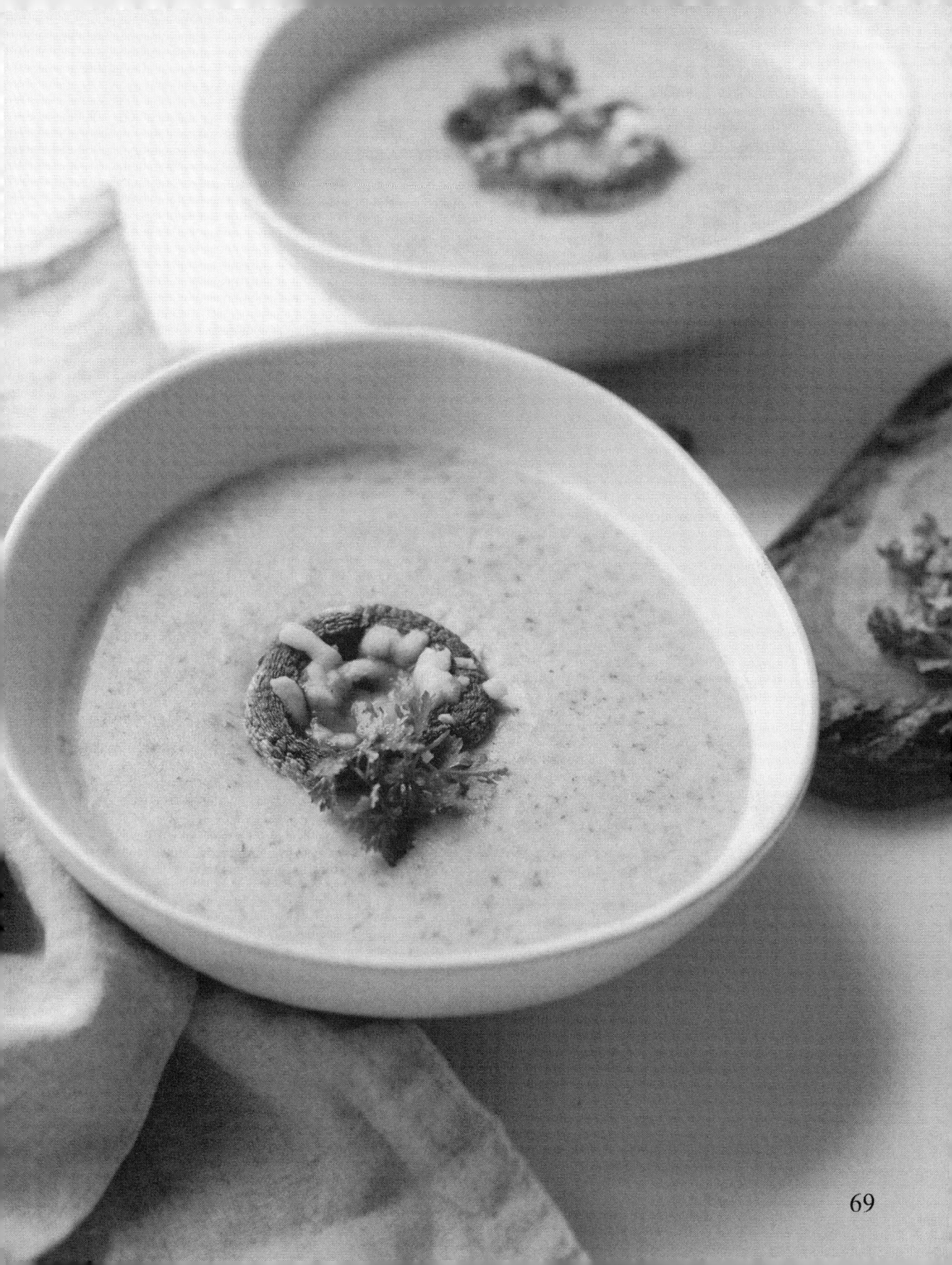

EASY GRILLED SHRIMP WITH AVOCADO AND TOMATO

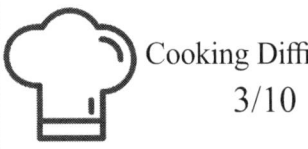 Cooking Difficulty: 3/10	 Cooking Time: 12 minutes	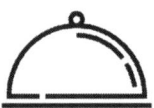 Servings: 6

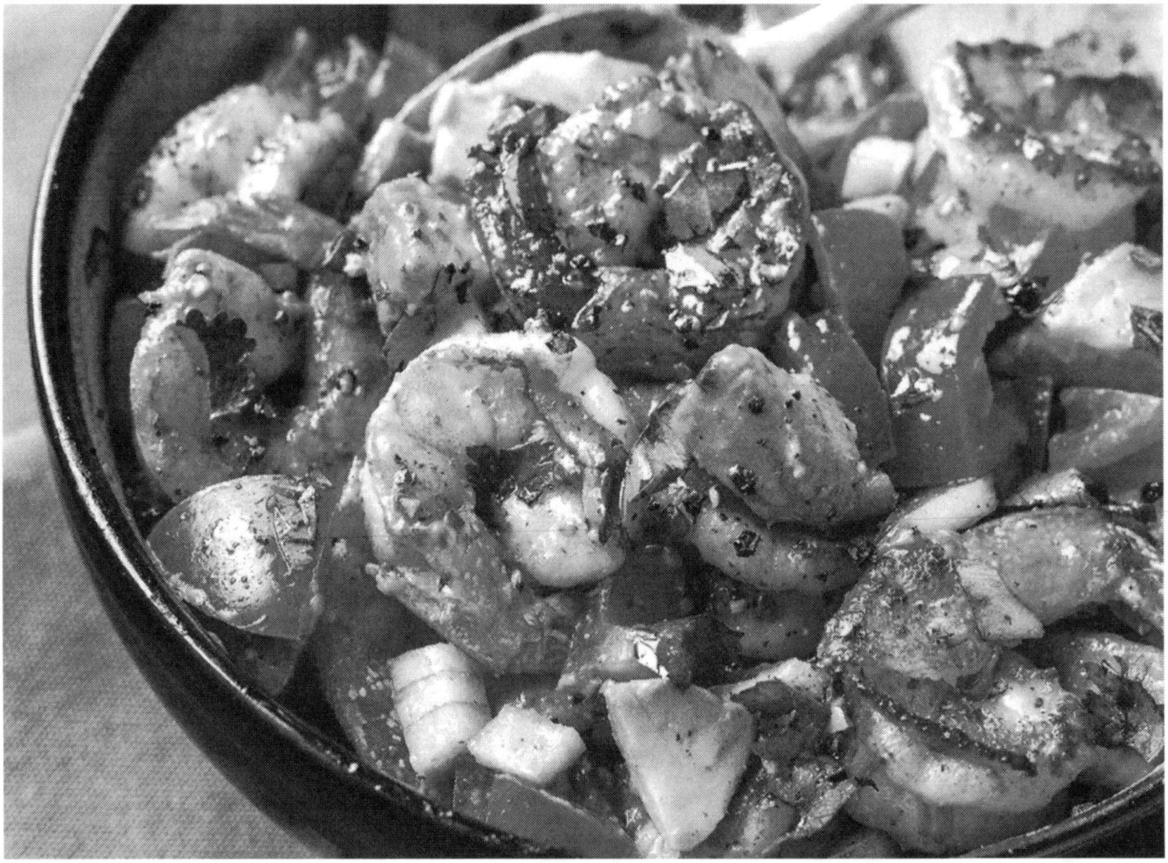

NUTRITIONAL INFORMATION

300 Calories, 11g Fats, 5g Carbs, 5g Protein

INGREDIENTS

- 2 cubed avocados
- 2 lb. deveined shrimp
- ½ c. chopped tomato
- ½ c. chopped bell pepper
- ½ c. chopped onion
- 4 tbsps. olive oil
- 2 tsps. squeezed lime juice
- 1 tsp. garlic powder
- 1 tsp. fine sea salt
- ¼ tsp. black pepper

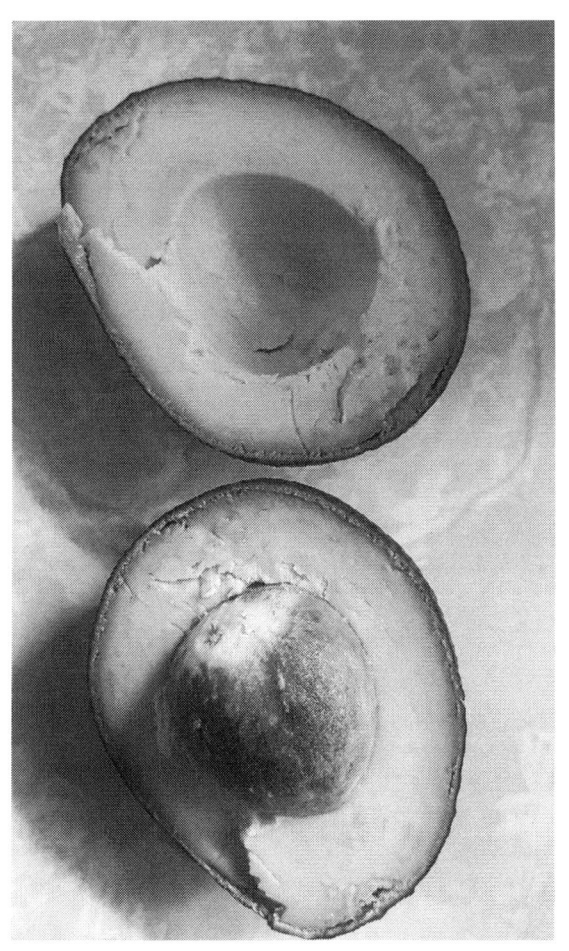

DESCRIPTION

STEP 1
Place a grill over medium-high flame and heat through.

STEP 2
Meanwhile, combine the garlic powder, half the salt and pepper, and olive oil in a large bowl. Add the shrimp and toss well to coat. Set aside.

STEP 3
In a salad bowl, combine the bell pepper, tomato, onion, avocado, and lime juice. Season with the remaining salt and toss gently to coat. Cover and refrigerate until ready to serve.

STEP 4
Cook the shrimp in the hot grill for 3 minutes per side, or until cooked through.

STEP 5
Divide the shrimp into individual servings, followed by the salad. Cover and refrigerate for up to 3 days. Reheat the shrimp before serving.

RADISH CUCUMBER SALAD

 Cooking Difficulty: 1/10

 Cooking Time: 3 minutes

 Servings: 2

INGREDIENTS

- 8 radishes
- 2 cucumber
- olive oil
- salt
- lime slice
- 0.5 cup fresh green peas
- salad greens

DESCRIPTION

STEP 1
Slice the radish and cucumber. Mix all ingredients, top with a lime slice on the salad and garnish with herbs as desired.

NUTRITIONAL INFORMATION

60 Calories, 0,4g Fats, 0,6g Carbs, and 0,2g Protein

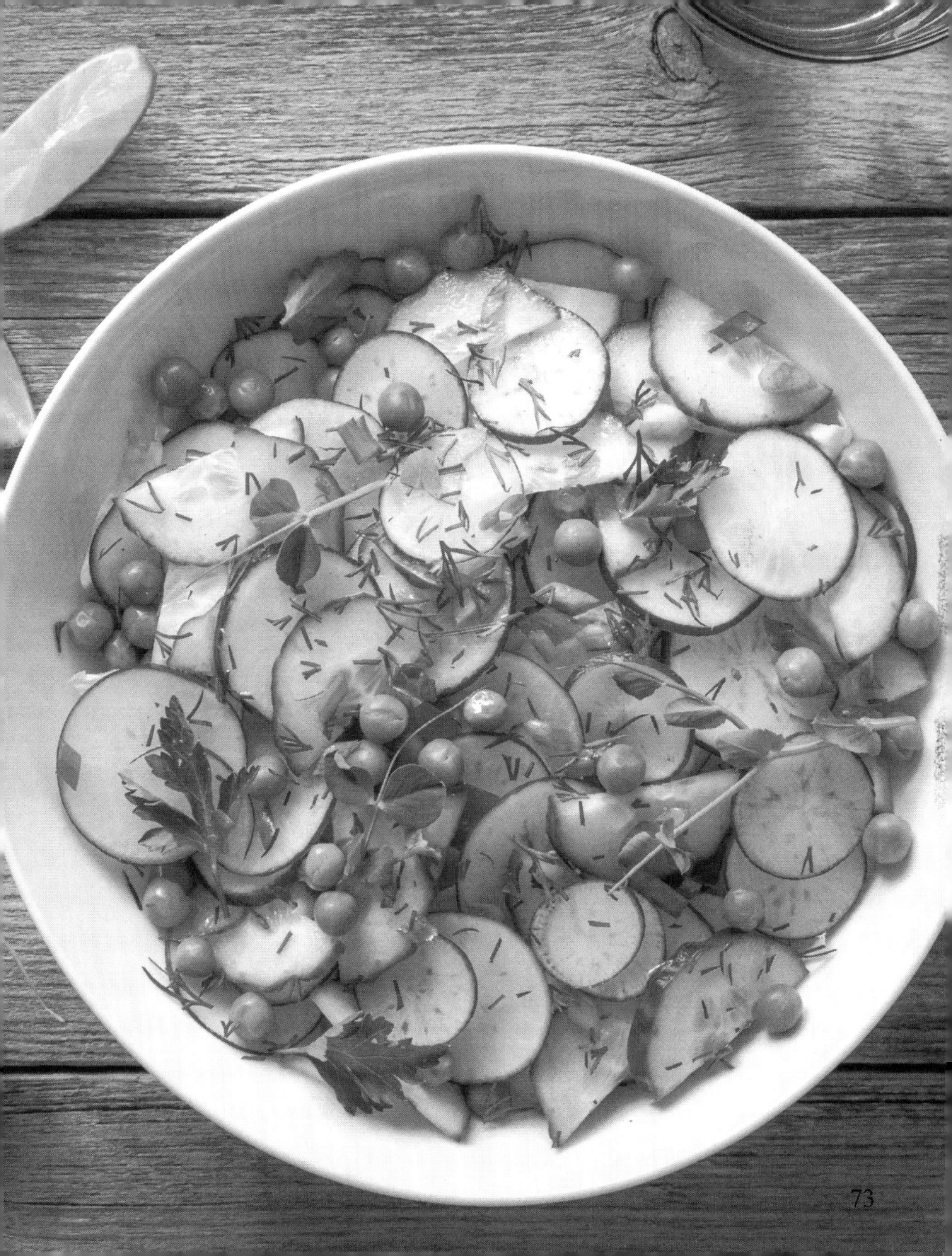

BAKED VEGETABLES

 Cooking Difficulty: 2/10

 Cooking Time: 35 minutes

 Servings: 2

INGREDIENTS

- 2 minced garlic cloves
- 2 tablespoons olive oil
- 1/2 pound broccoli florets
- 2 carrots
- green beans (optional)
- black pepper
- salt
- 2 eggs

DESCRIPTION

STEP 1
Slice the carrots into slices. In a roasting pan, combine the vegetables together with the oil, garlic and spices, toss and bake at 400 degrees F for 15 minutes.

STEP 2
When the time is up, take out the mold and pour the two eggs into it. Return to the oven and bake until the eggs are cooked.

STEP 3
Divide the mix between plates and serve.

NUTRITIONAL INFORMATION

260 Calories, 4.9g Protein, 7g Fat, 4,4g Carbs

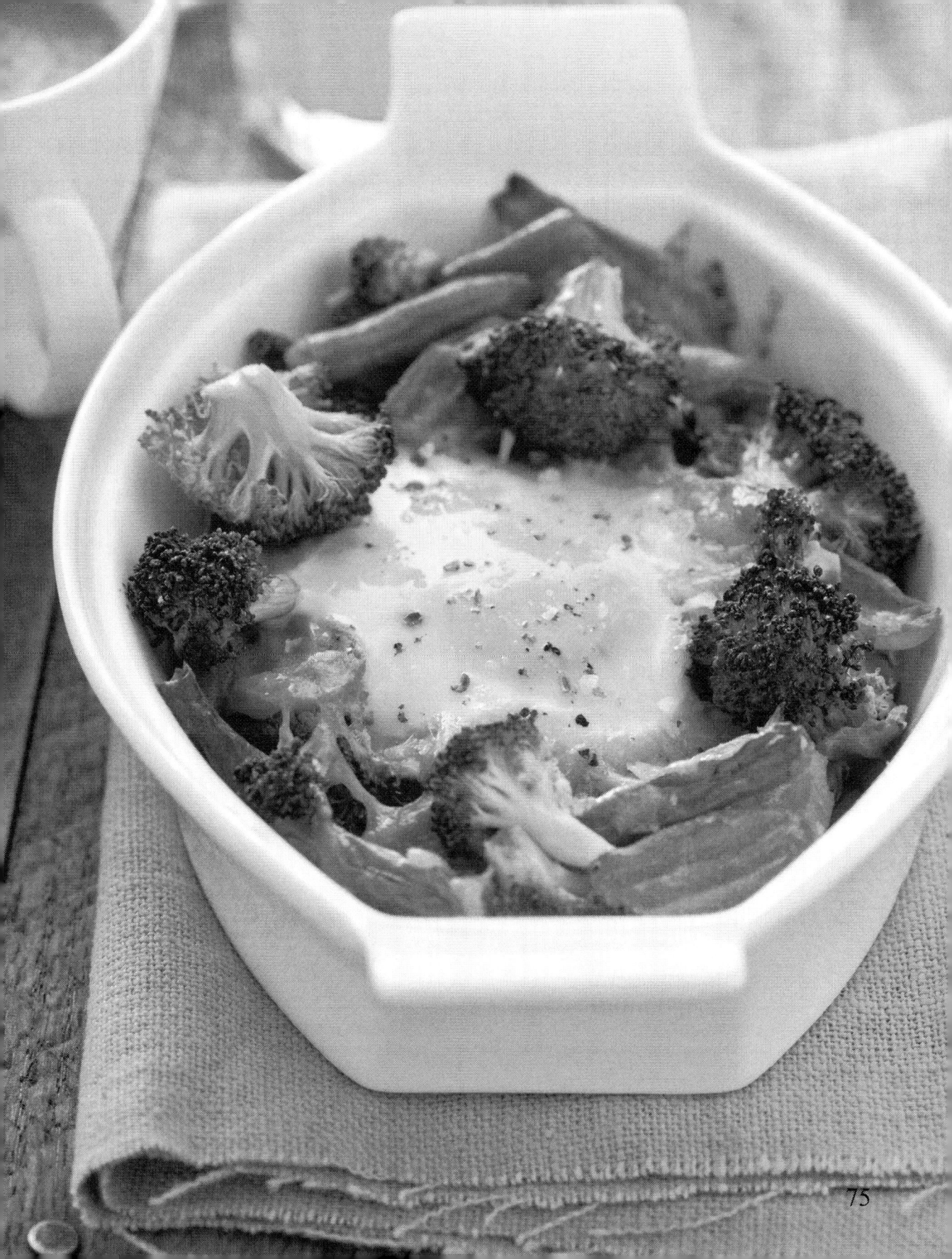

ITALIAN TOMATO SOUP

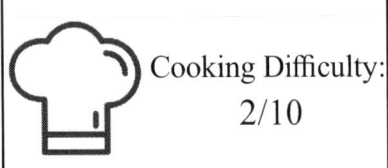 Cooking Difficulty:
2/10

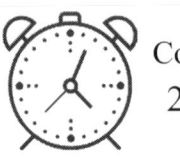 Cooking Time:
25 minutes

 Servings:
3

INGREDIENTS

- 1 pound tomatoes
- 3 cloves of garlic
- 3 cups vegetable broth
- 2 tbsp. olive oil
- 1 green basil, bundle
- dry bread (optional)
- sea salt
- black pepper

DESCRIPTION

STEP 1
Heat olive oil in a large saucepan over medium heat. Add the garlic and fry for 1 minute.

STEP 2
In a separate bowl, chop the tomatoes. Place them in the pan. Season with salt and pepper. Partially cover and stew over medium heat for about ten minutes. Add the broth and basil, return to the stove and simmer for another ten minutes. Add the bread cubes and stew for another ten minutes until the bread is soft.

STEP 3
Serve with extra olive oil and put in more fresh basil!

NUTRITIONAL INFORMATION

110 Calories, 2g Fats, 3g Carbs, and 3g Protein

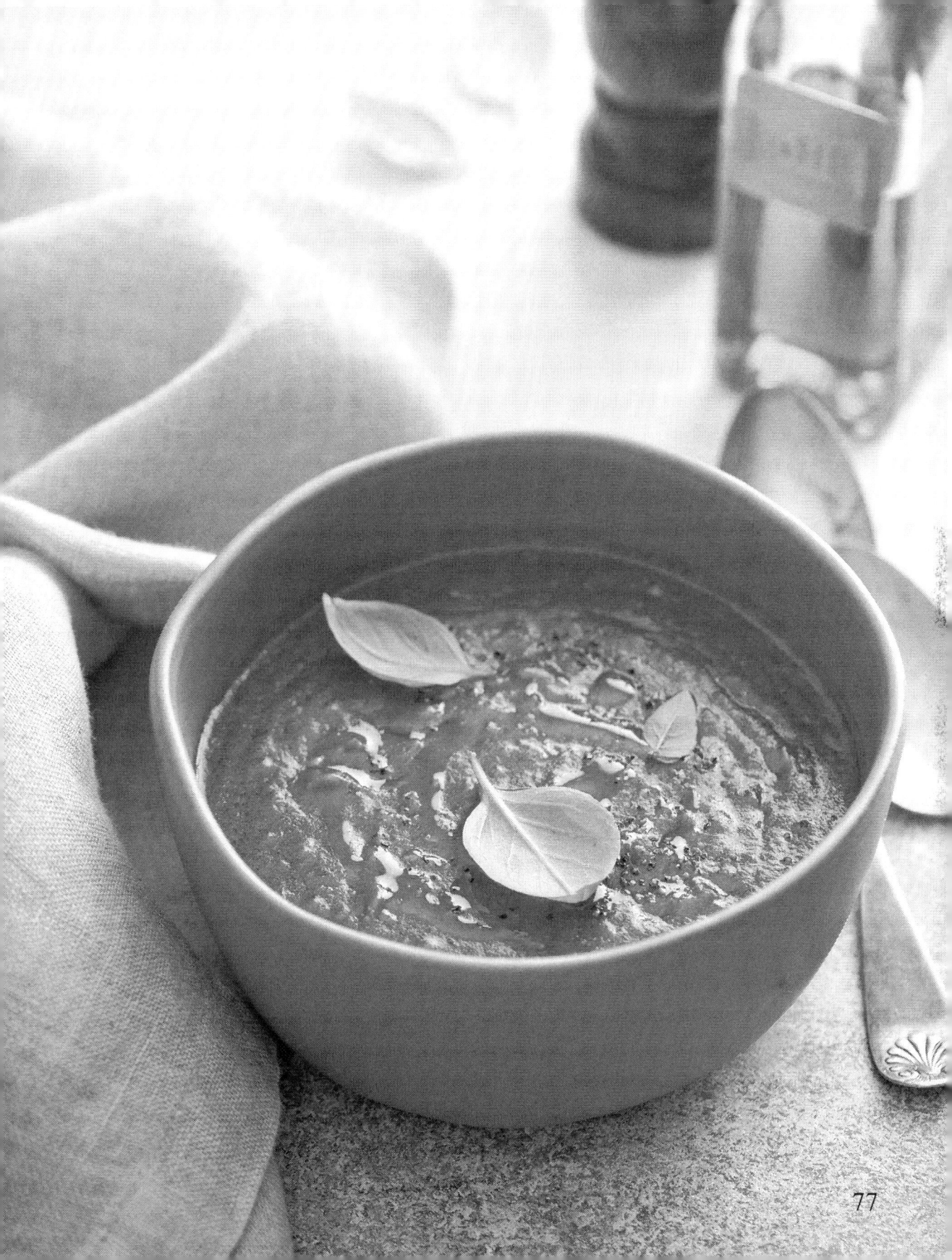

GARLIC SHRIMP

 Cooking Difficulty:
1/10

 Cooking Time:
15 minutes

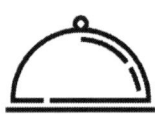 Servings:
4

INGREDIENTS

- 2 pounds of peeled shrimp
- salt
- pepper
- 4 cloves garlic
- lemon
- olive oil

DESCRIPTION

STEP 1
Mix garlic, spices and oil together.

STEP 2
Wash shrimp and dip each one in garlic oil.

STEP 3
Drizzle the shrimp with lemon juice and fry for 4 minutes on each side.

STEP 4
Serve hot.

NUTRITIONAL INFORMATION

210 Calories, 7g Fats, 4g Carbs, and 4g Protein

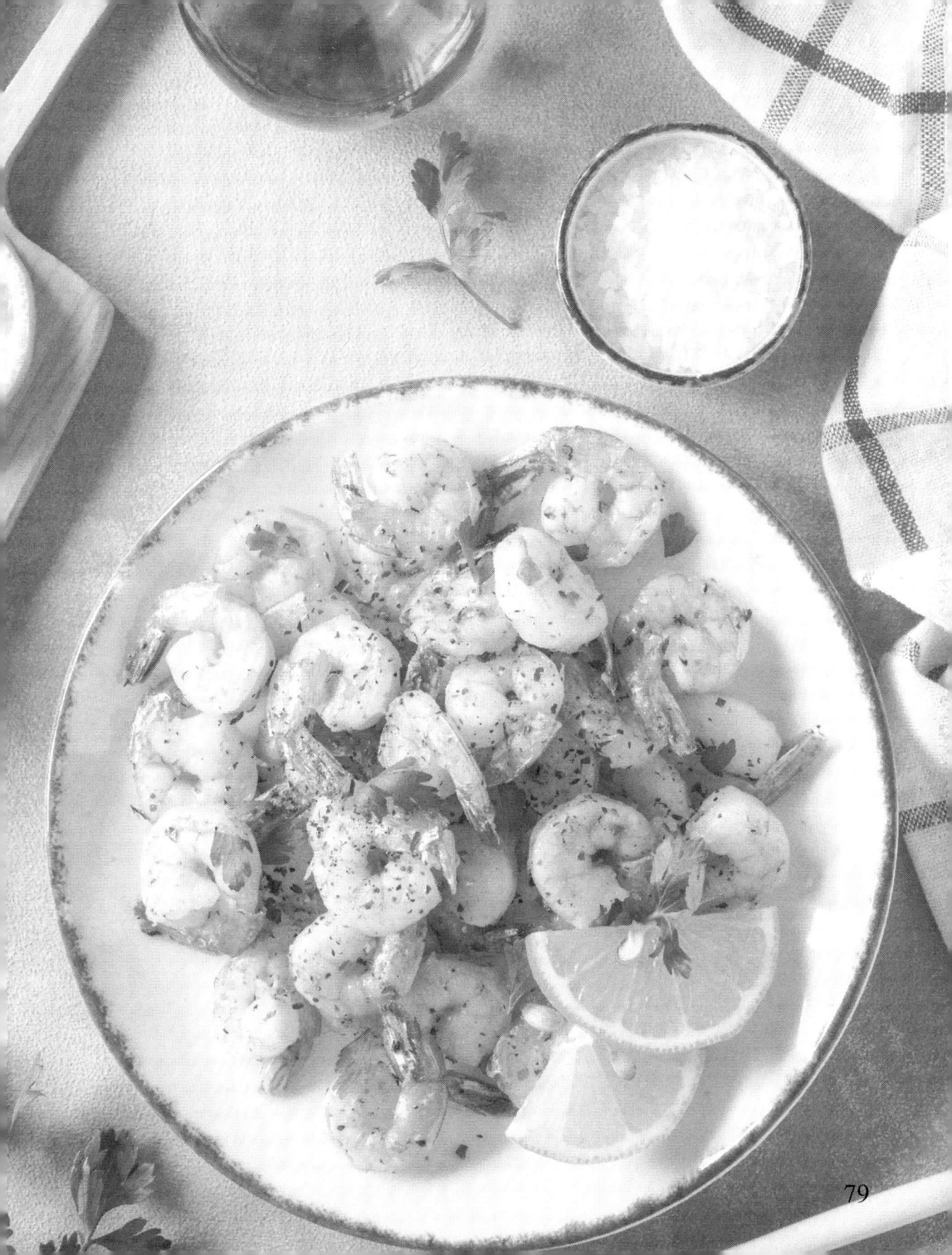

SHRIMP AND STRAWBERRY SALAD

 Cooking Difficulty: 2/10	 Cooking Time: 5 minutes	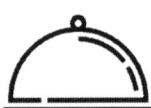 Servings: 4

INGREDIENTS

- 2 tbsps. balsamic vinegar
- 2 c. strawberries halved
- 1 c. baby spinach
- 1 tbsp. lemon juice
- 2 garlic cloves, minced
- 1 lb. shrimp, peeled and deveined
- 2 tbsps. olive oil
- favorite seeds as desired

DESCRIPTION

STEP 1
Heat up a pan with the oil over medium-high heat, add the garlic, and brown for 1 minute.

STEP 2
Add the shrimp and lemon juice, toss, and cook for 3 minutes on each side.

STEP 3
In a salad bowl, combine the shrimp and the other ingredients, toss, and serve for lunch.

NUTRITIONAL INFORMATION

Calories 260, Fat 9.7g, Carbs 16.5g, Protein 28g

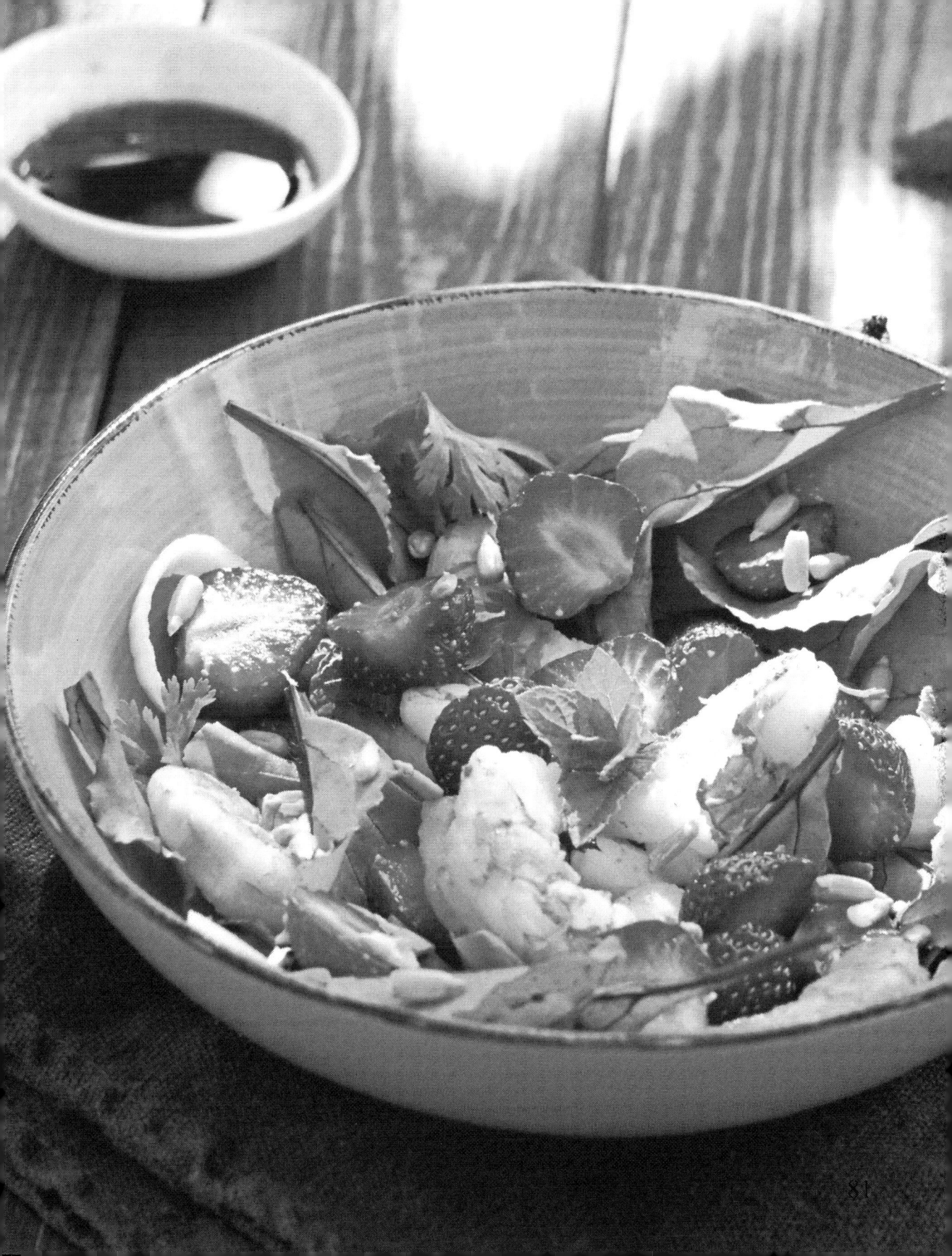

PASTA WITH BROCCOLI

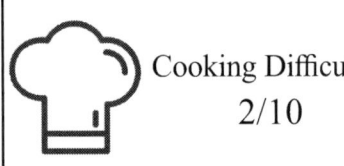 Cooking Difficulty: 2/10

 Cooking Time: 20 minutes

 Servings: 3

INGREDIENTS

- 8 ounces (225g) whole wheat or whole grain pasta
- 2 cups broccoli florets
- 2 tablespoons olive oil
  3 cloves garlic, minced
- 1/4 teaspoon red pepper flakes (optional, for a spicy kick)
- Salt and pepper to taste

DESCRIPTION

STEP 1
Boil 8 oz (225 g) whole-grain pasta in salted water until al dente. Prepare 2 cups of broccoli florets.

STEP 2
In a large skillet, heat 2 tablespoons olive oil and fry 3 garlic cloves, minced, over medium heat for about 1 minute. Add the broccoli and stir. Salt and pepper to taste.

STEP 3
Add the boiled pasta to the skillet and stir well so that the pasta and broccoli are evenly coated with the sauce.

NUTRITIONAL INFORMATION

260 Calories, 4.9g Protein, 7g Fat, 4,4g Carbs

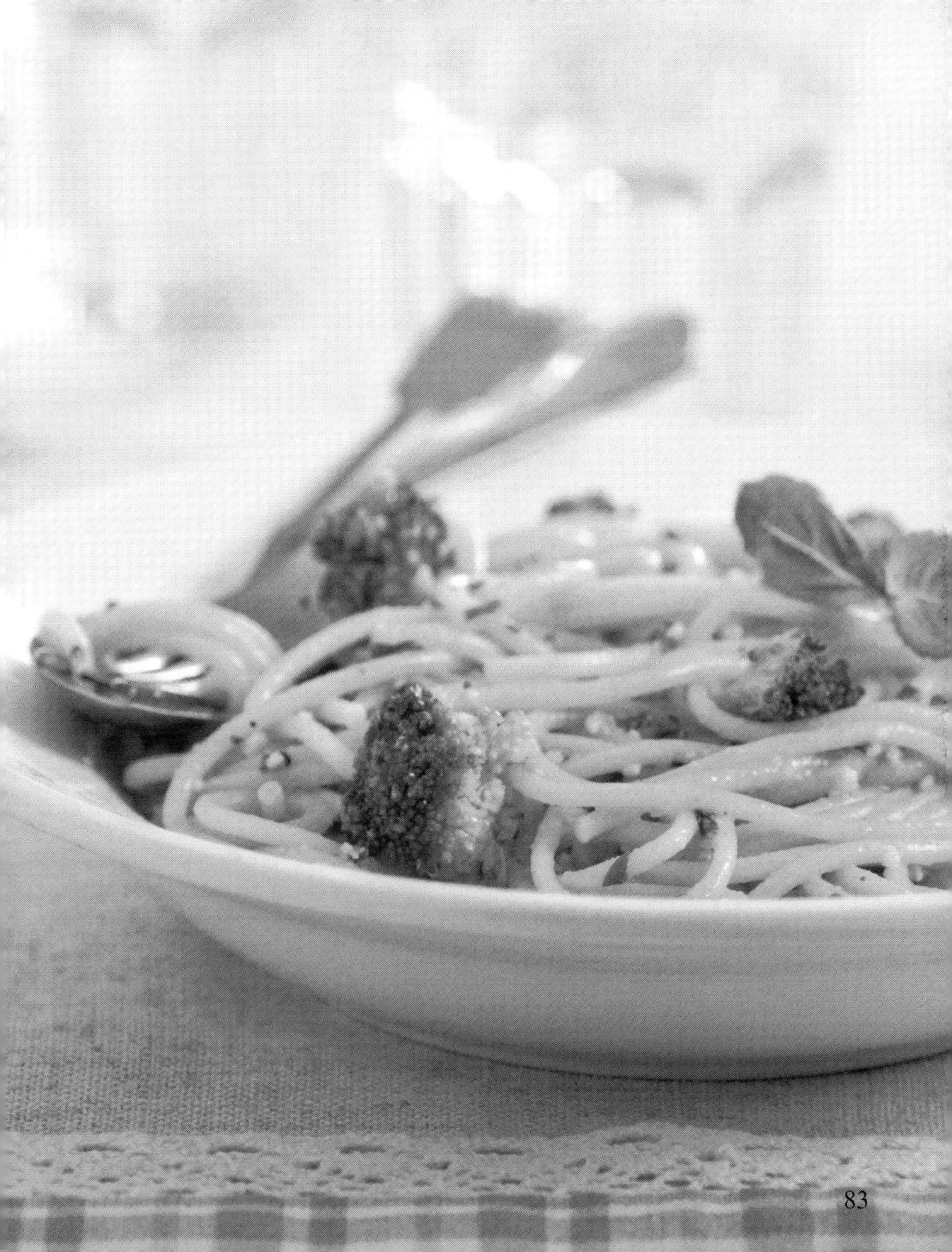

QUINOA WITH ACORN SQUASH & SWISS CHARD

 Cooking Difficulty: 2/10	 Cooking Time: 7 minutes	 Servings: 4

INGREDIENTS

- ¾ c. canned acorn squash puree
- ½ tbsp. moroccan seasoning
- 1¾ c. uncooked quinoa, well rinsed
- ½ tsp. sea salt
- 2½ c. water
- ¼ tsp. ground allspice
- 1½ c. swiss chard, trimmed and torn into pieces

DESCRIPTION

STEP 1
Throw all the ingredients into the pot except for the Swiss chard.

STEP 2
Set the pot to Manual mode, on high, with a cook time of 5-minutes.

STEP 3
When the cooking time is completed, release the pressure using quick-release.

STEP 4
Add the Swiss chard and stir, serve right away.

NUTRITIONAL INFORMATION

Calories: 281, Fat: 4.6g, Carbs: 23g, Protein: 12.1g

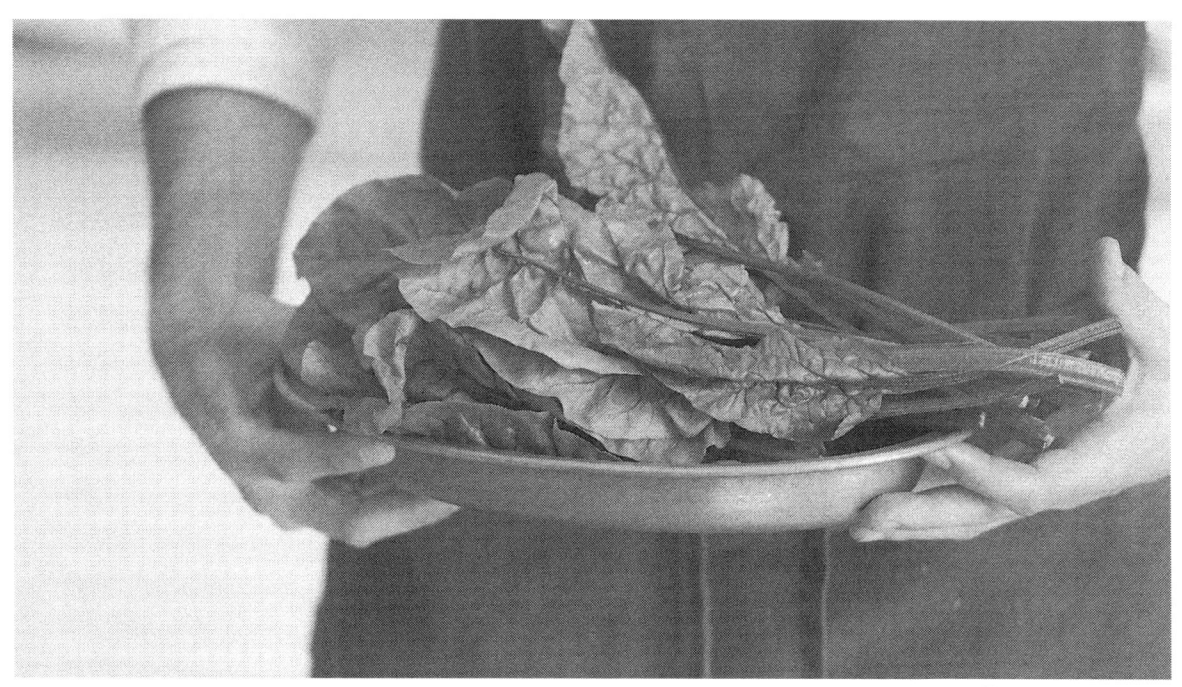

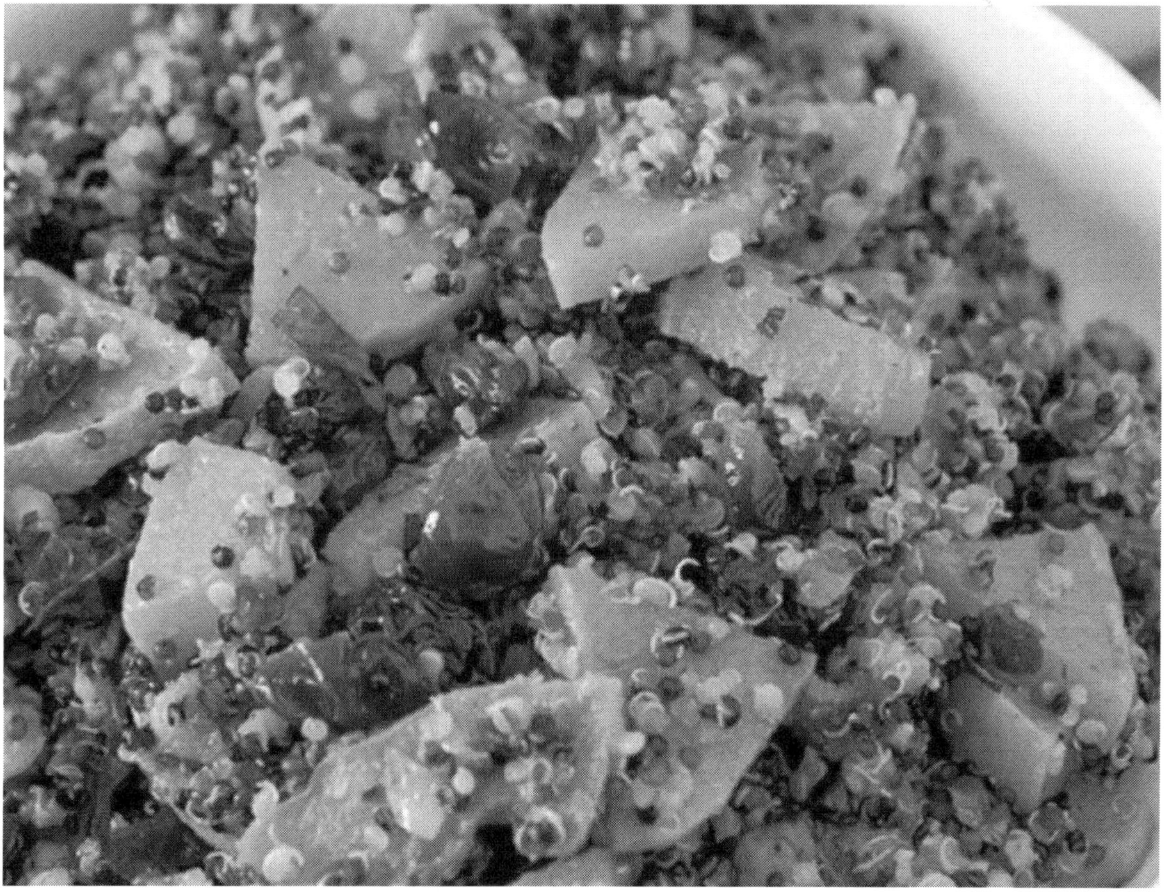

CHICKEN COUSCOUS

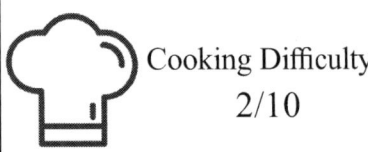 Cooking Difficulty: 2/10

 Cooking Time: 17 minutes

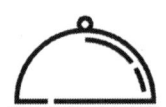 Servings: 8

INGREDIENTS

- 3 c. chopped chicken
- 1 ¼ c. chicken broth
- 1 pint grape tomatoes
- 1 tsp. lemon rind
- 1 5.6 oz. package of toasted pine nut couscous mix
- ¼ c. chopped fresh basil
- ¼ tsp. pepper
- salt

DESCRIPTION

STEP 1
You will want to begin this by heating the chicken broth and the seasoning packet from the couscous in a microwave for three to five minutes while on high.

STEP 2
Once the broth is boiling, mix it with the couscous in a large bowl and allow it to stand for about five minutes. Once the time has passed, fluff the couscous with a fork and stir in the chicken.

STEP 4
When this is complete, mix in your spices and vegetables. Your meal is complete!

NUTRITIONAL INFORMATION

334 Calories, 10.9g Fat, 35.8g Carbs, 20.9g Protein

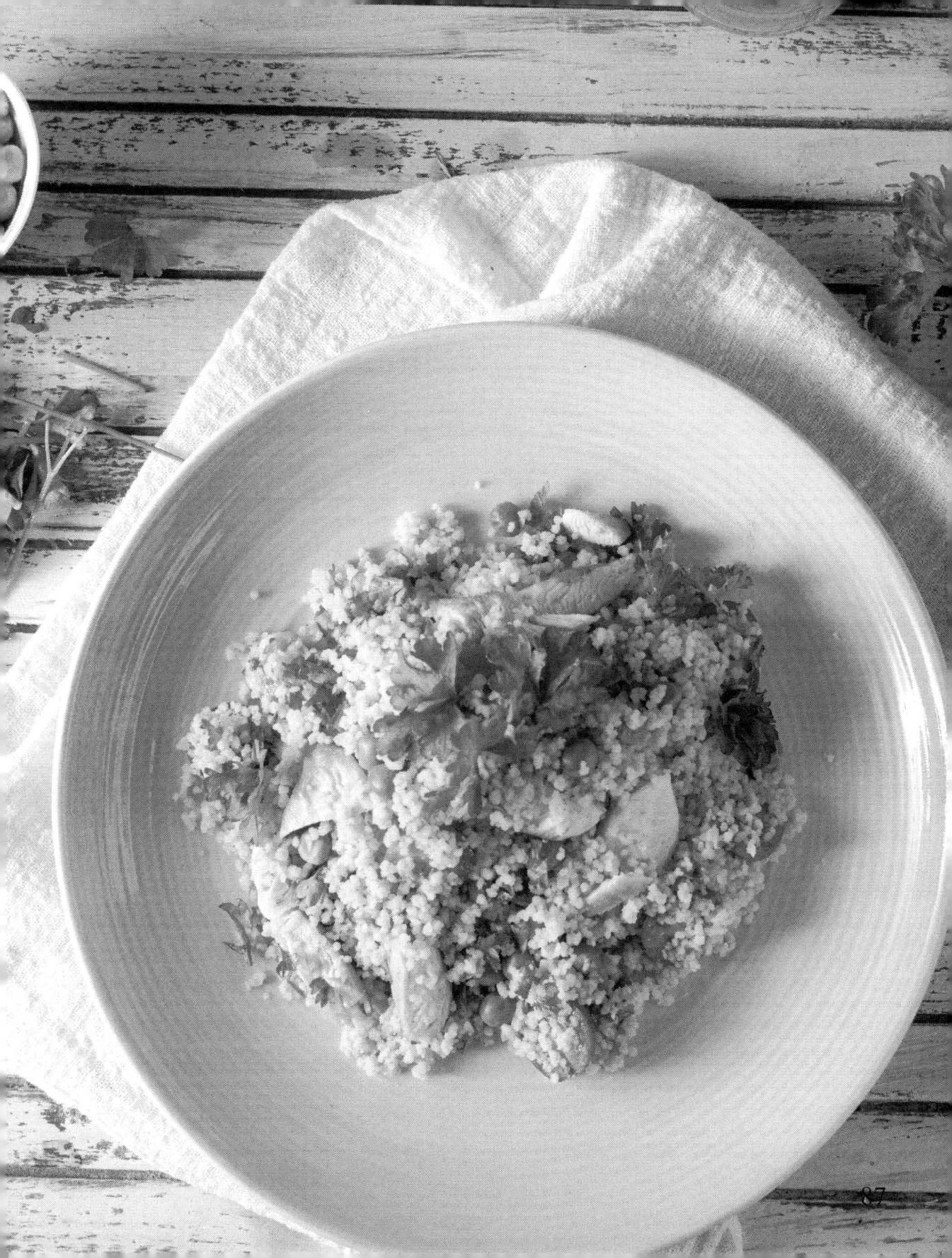

RADISH SALMON SALAD

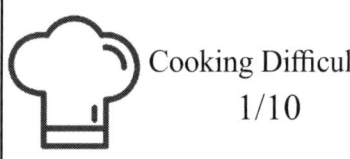 Cooking Difficulty: 1/10

 Cooking Time: 3 minutes

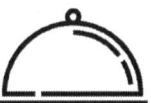 Servings: 2

INGREDIENTS

- 1 grilled and sliced salmon steak
- 2 tablespoons olive oil
- 8 sliced radishes
- 2 tbsp. lemon juice
- black pepper
- salt
- favorite lettuce leaves

DESCRIPTION

STEP 1
In a bowl, mix the radishes slices with the salmon and the rest of the ingredients, stir and serve for lunch.

NUTRITIONAL INFORMATION

Calories 300, Fat 8g, Carbs 5g, Protein 6g

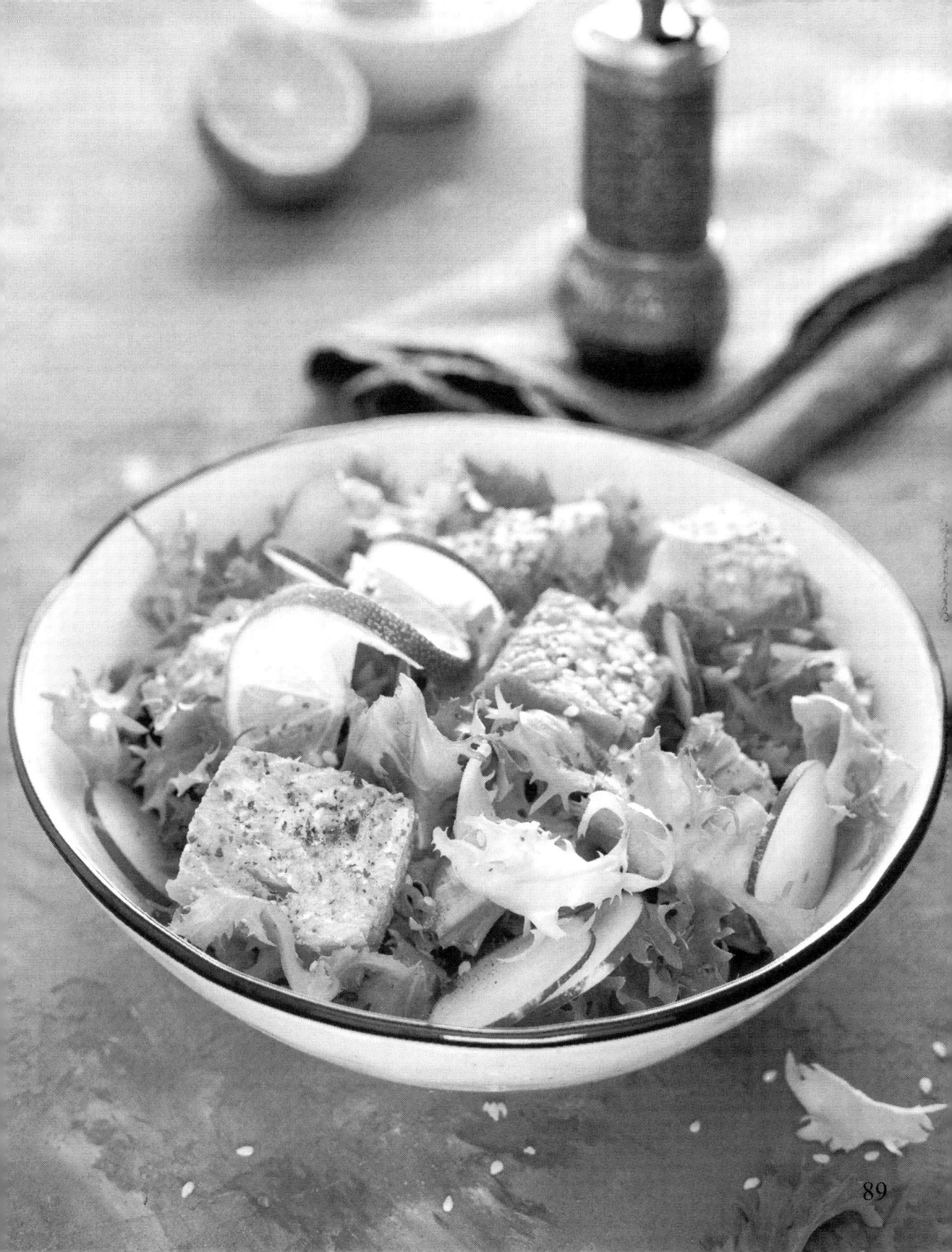

SHRIMP SALAD

 Cooking Difficulty: 2/10	 Cooking Time: 8 minutes	 Servings: 4

INGREDIENTS

- 1 lb. shrimp, deveined and peeled
- 1 onion, sliced
- ¼ tsp. black pepper
- 2 c. baby arugula
- 1 tbsp. lemon juice
- 1 tbsp. avocado or olive oil
- pine nuts

DESCRIPTION

STEP 1
Heat up a pan with the oil over medium heat, add the onion, stir, and sauté for 2 minutes.

STEP 2
Add the shrimp and cook for 6 minutes. Mix all the ingredients, divide into bowls, and serve.

NUTRITIONAL INFORMATION

Calories 341, Fat 11.5g, Carbs 17.3g, Protein 14.3g

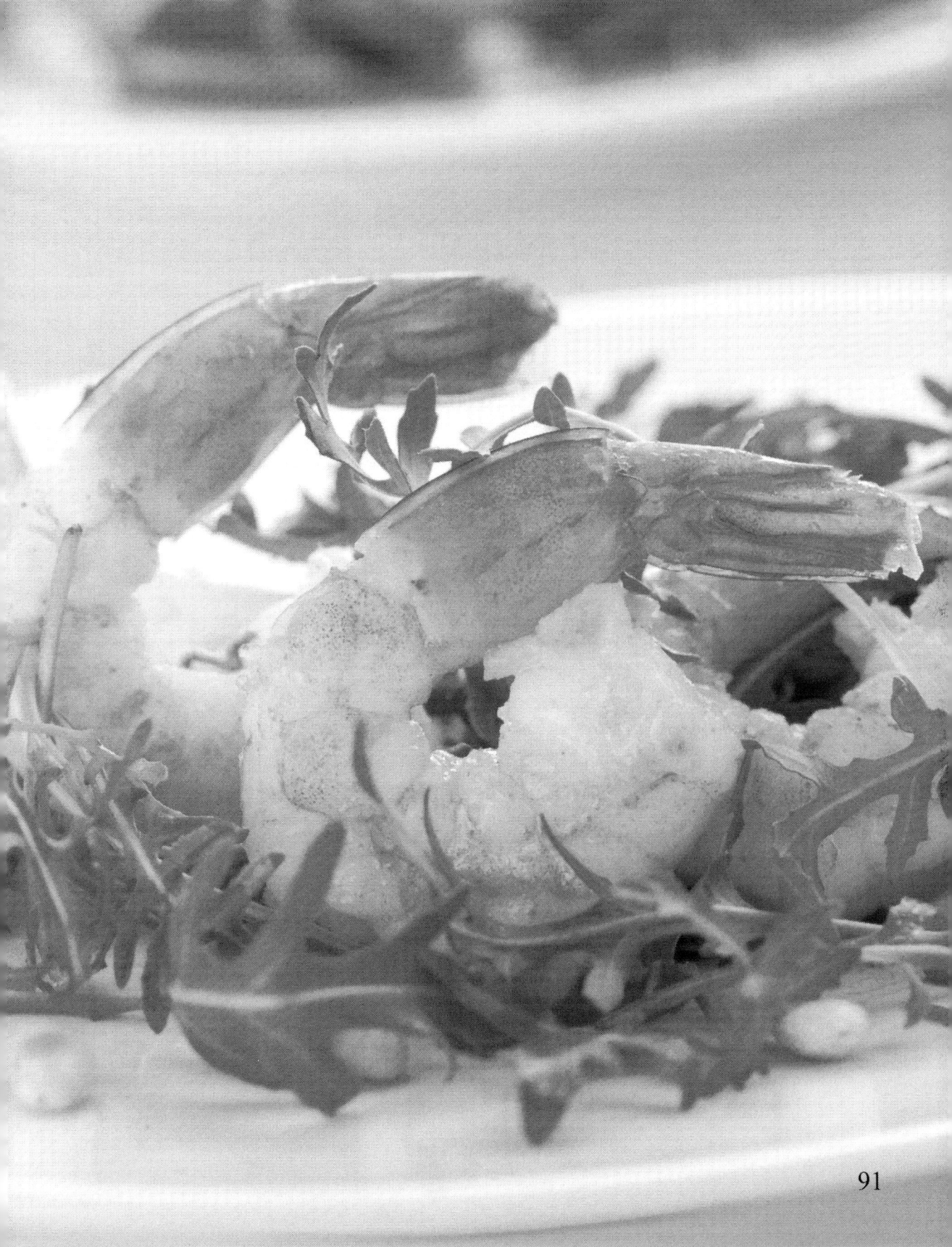

AVOCADO SALMON SALAD

 Cooking Difficulty: 1/10

 Cooking Time: 3 minutes

 Servings: 2

INGREDIENTS

- chopped lightly salted salmon
- 2 tbsp. avocado oil
- 2 sliced avocados
- 2 tbsp. lime juice
- 1 sliced cucumber
- black pepper
- favorite lettuce leaves if desired

DESCRIPTION

STEP 1

In a bowl, mix the avocado slices with the salmon and the rest of the ingredients, stir and serve for lunch.

NUTRITIONAL INFORMATION

Calories 200, Fat 10g, Carbs 3g, Protein 7g

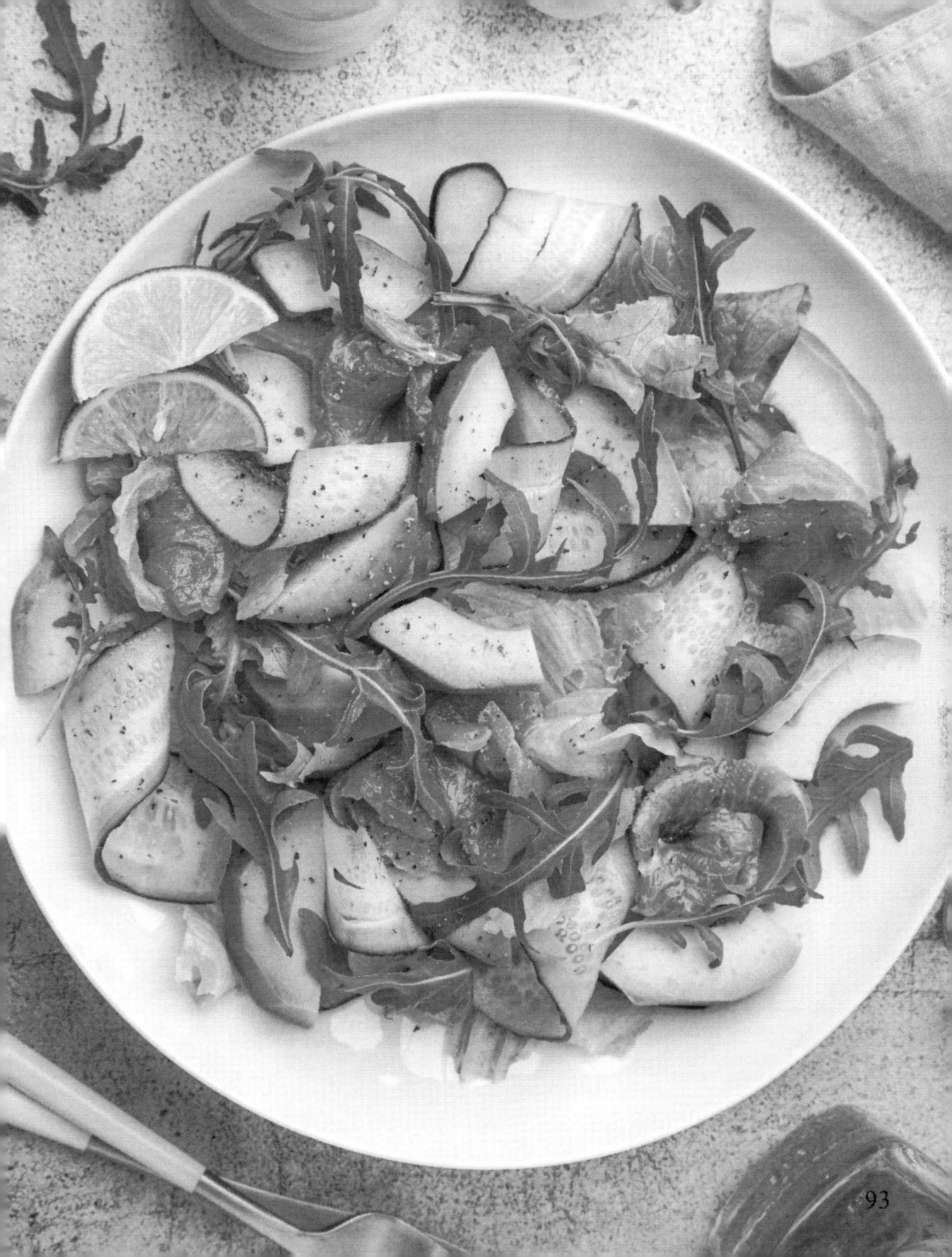

ZUCCHINI CAKES

 Cooking Difficulty: 2/10

 Cooking Time: 22 minutes

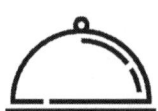 Servings: 4

INGREDIENTS

- 2 tbsps. olive oil
- 2 tbsps. almond flour
- 1/3 c. carrot, shredded
- 1 tsp. lemon zest, grated
- 1 garlic clove, minced
- 1 egg, whisked
- 2 zucchinis, grated
- 1 yellow onion, chopped
- black pepper
- sea salt

DESCRIPTION

STEP 1

In a bowl, combine the zucchinis with the garlic, onion, and the other ingredients except for the oil, stir well and shape medium cakes out of this mix.

STEP 2

Heat up a pan with the oil over medium-high heat, add the zucchini cakes, cook for 5 minutes on each side, divide between plates and serve with a side salad.

NUTRITIONAL INFORMATION

Calories 271, Fat 8.7g, Carbs 14.3g, Protein 4.6g

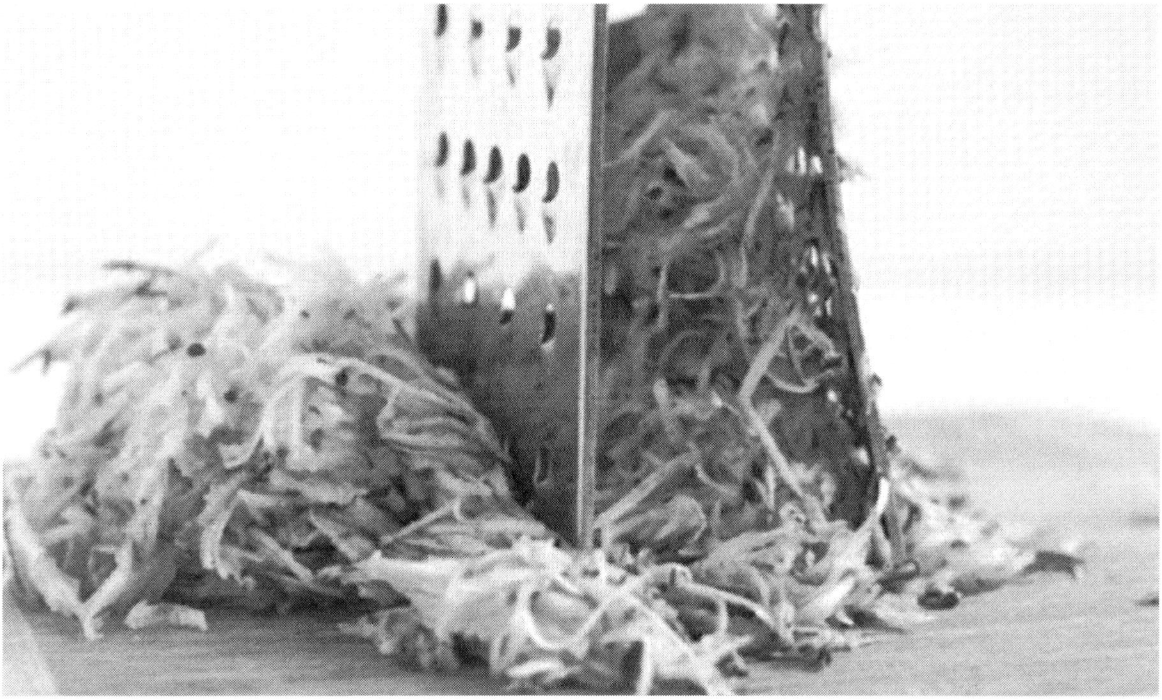

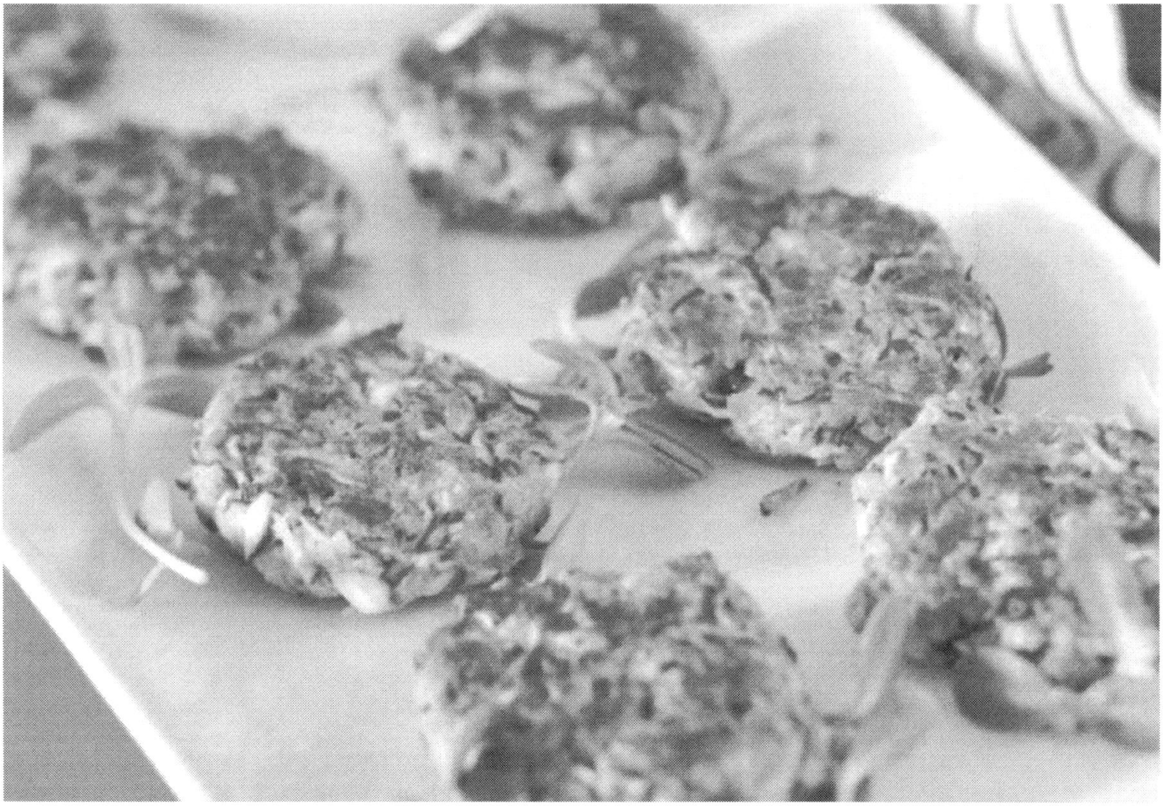

BLACK BEAN AND QUINOA SALAD

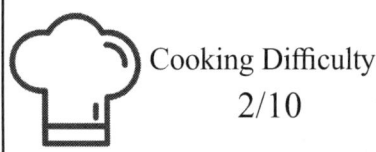 Cooking Difficulty: 2/10	 Cooking Time: 5 minutes	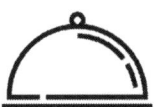 Servings: 10

INGREDIENTS

- 15 ounces boiled black beans
- 1 chopped red bell pepper without core
- 1 in. quinoa, cooked
- 1 green bell pepper, cored, chopped
- 5 ounces of canned corn
- parsley

DESCRIPTION

STEP 1
In a bowl, set in all ingredients, and stir until incorporated.

STEP 2
Top the salad with parsley and serve straight away. Place remaining portions in an airtight container and refrigerate for up to 4 days.

NUTRITIONAL INFORMATION

Calories: 64, Fat: 1 g, Carbs: 8 g, Protein: 3 g

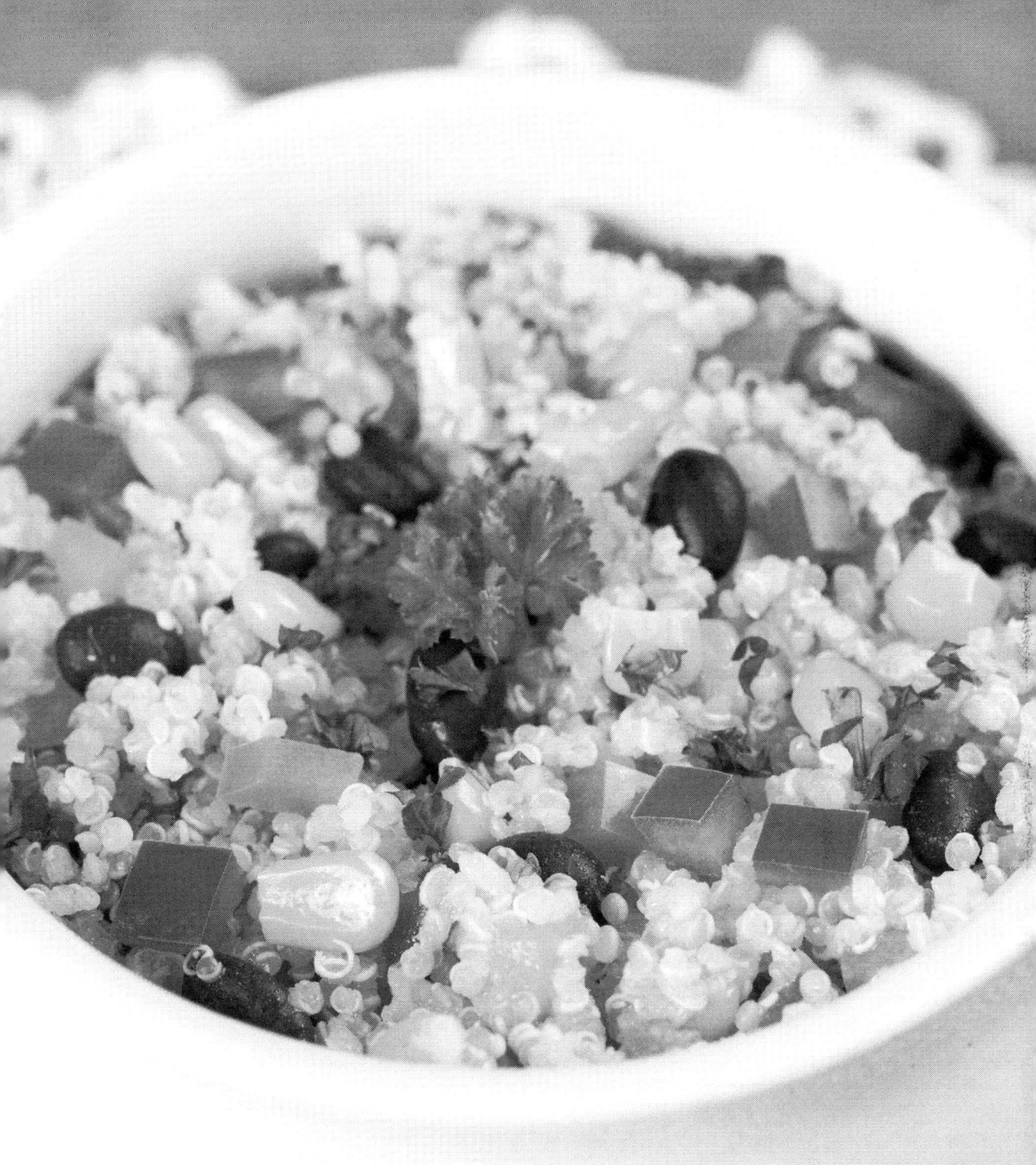

CAULIFLOWER AND GREEN BEANS

 Cooking Difficulty: 2/10

 Cooking Time: 30 minutes

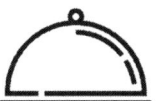 Servings: 4

INGREDIENTS

- 1 lb. cauliflower florets
- 1 tbsp. olive oil
- 2 minced garlic cloves
- 1 c. tomato pasta
- salt
- black pepper
- ½ lb. trimmed green beans halved
- 1 tbsp. chopped cilantro
- green peas optional

DESCRIPTION

STEP 1
Heat up a pot with the oil over medium-high heat; add the garlic and sauté for 3 minutes.

STEP 2
Add the cauliflower and the other ingredients, toss, then cook everything for 25 minutes more.

STEP 2
Divide everything between plates and serve.

NUTRITIONAL INFORMATION

Calories 93, Fat 3.7g, Carbs 13.7g, Protein 4.1g

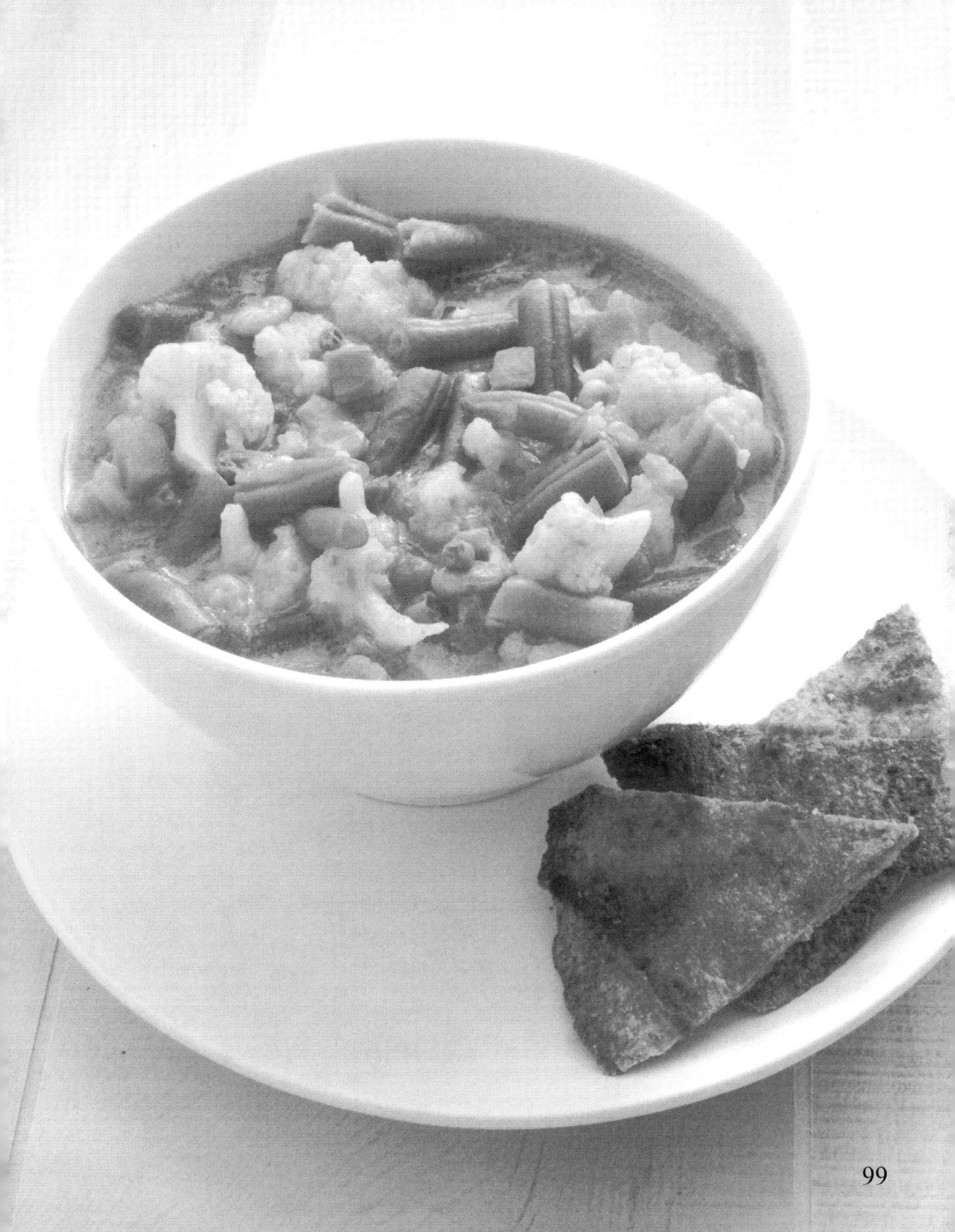

CAULIFLOWER WITH SAUSAGE AND LEEKS TOPPINGS

 Cooking Difficulty: 3/10	 Cooking Time: 26 minutes	 Servings: 6

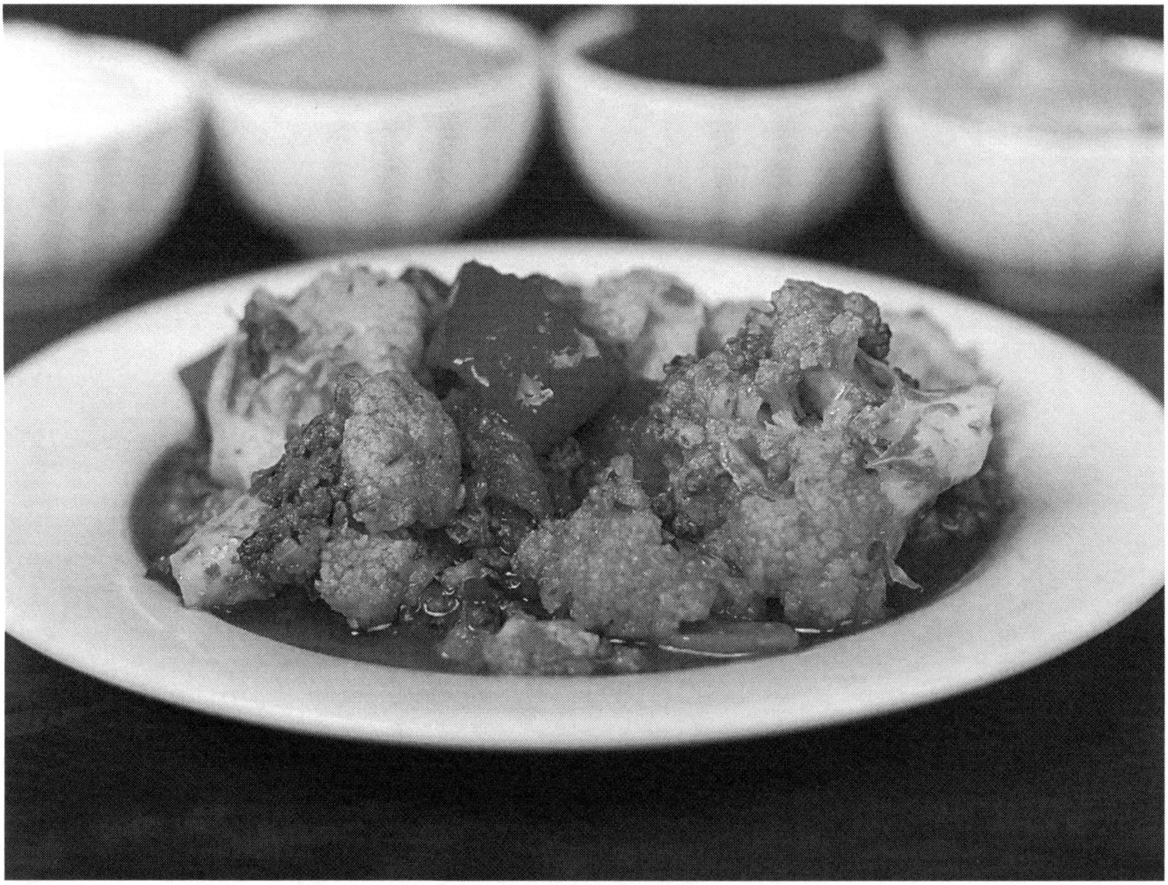

NUTRITIONAL INFORMATION

258 Calories, 18g Carbs, 7g Protein, 10g Fat

INGREDIENTS

- 28 oz. crushed tomatoes
- 1 cauliflower head
- 1 lb. ground sausage
- ½ tsp. granulated garlic
- ½ tsp. red pepper flakes (optional)
- 2 tbsps. italian seasoning
- 2 tsps. himalayan pink salt
- 3 medium chopped leeks
- ½ lemon

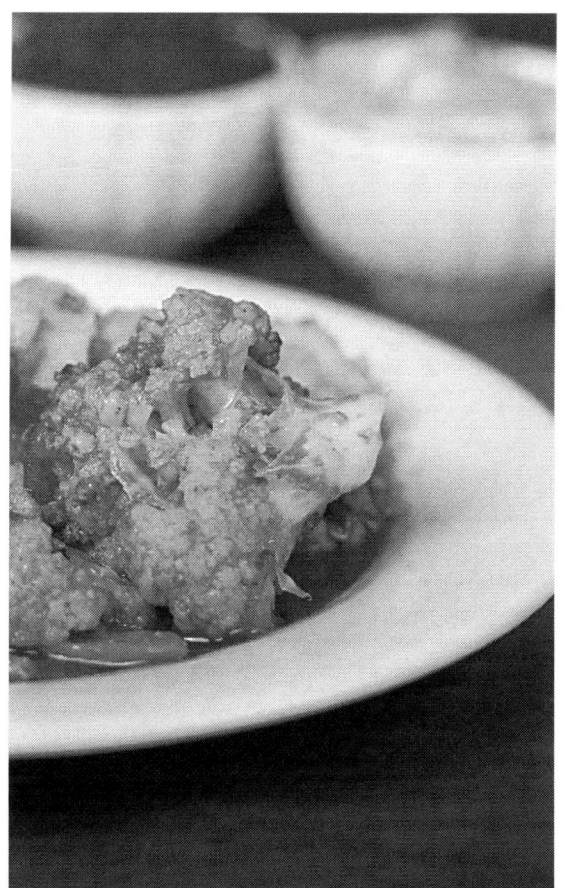

DESCRIPTION

STEP 1
Over med-high heat, heat a 3 to 4-quart pan. Add leeks and butter and sauté for 3 to 5 mins.

STEP 2
Add sausage and cook with frequent stirring until the meat is cooked through.

STEP 3
Add Italian seasoning, lemon, tomatoes, granulated garlic, and red pepper flakes. Simmer over medium heat for 20 mins. And stir occasionally.

STEP 4
While waiting, microwave the cauliflower for 5 mins.

STEP 5
Add Himalayan pink salt to season the tomato sauce and sausage and serve over the cauliflower.

TUNA SALAD WITH AVOCADO

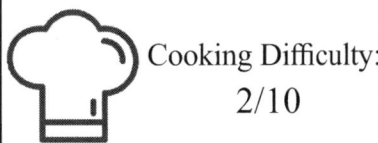 Cooking Difficulty: 2/10

 Cooking Time: 5 minutes

 Servings: 3

INGREDIENTS

- 1 ripe avocado
- ½ tsp. lemon juice
- ¼ tsp. mustard
- 4 oz. wild tuna
- garlic powder
- onion powder
- parsley flakes
- 2 tomoto (optional)
- black pepper

DESCRIPTION

STEP 1
Slice the avocado and mash it in a bowl and add tuna.

STEP 2
Season with garlic powder, parsley, onion powder, lemon juice and mustard.

STEP 3
Rip off lettuce leaves and add a spoonful of avocado mixture in each leaf. Eat using your hands and enjoy.

NUTRITIONAL INFORMATION

Calories 271, Fat 8.7g, Carbs 14.3g, Protein 4.6g

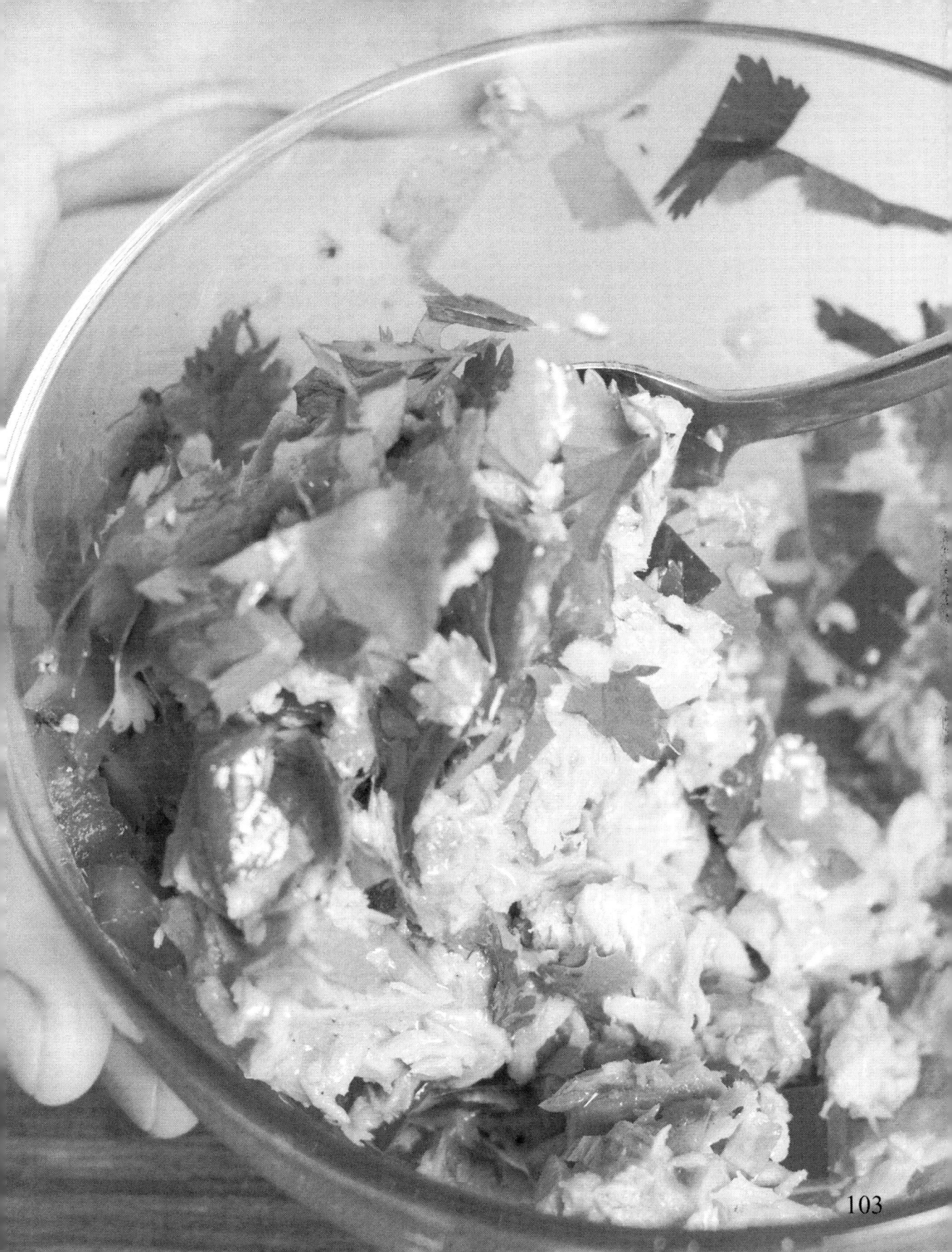

BAKED BROCCOLI

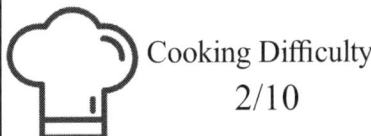 Cooking Difficulty: 2/10

 Cooking Time: 20 minutes

 Servings: 4

INGREDIENTS

- 2 minced garlic cloves
- 2 tbsps. olive oil
- 1 lb. broccoli florets
- ½ tsp. ground nutmeg
- black pepper

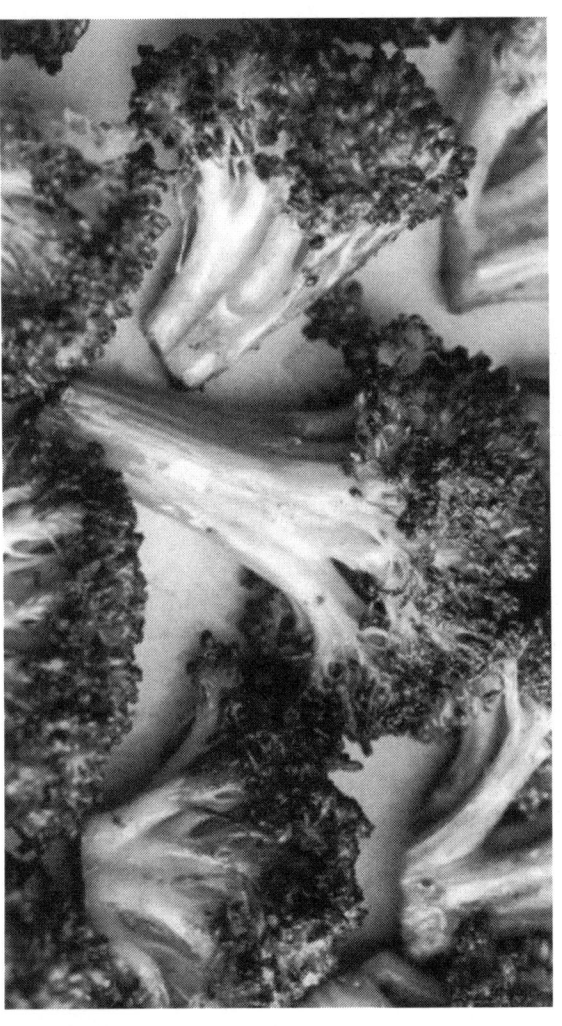

DESCRIPTION

STEP 1

In a roasting pan, combine the broccoli with the garlic and the other ingredients, toss and bake at 400 degrees F for 20 minutes.

STEP 2

Divide the mix between plates and serve.

NUTRITIONAL INFORMATION

365 Calories, 22g Fats, 7g Carbs, 7g Protein

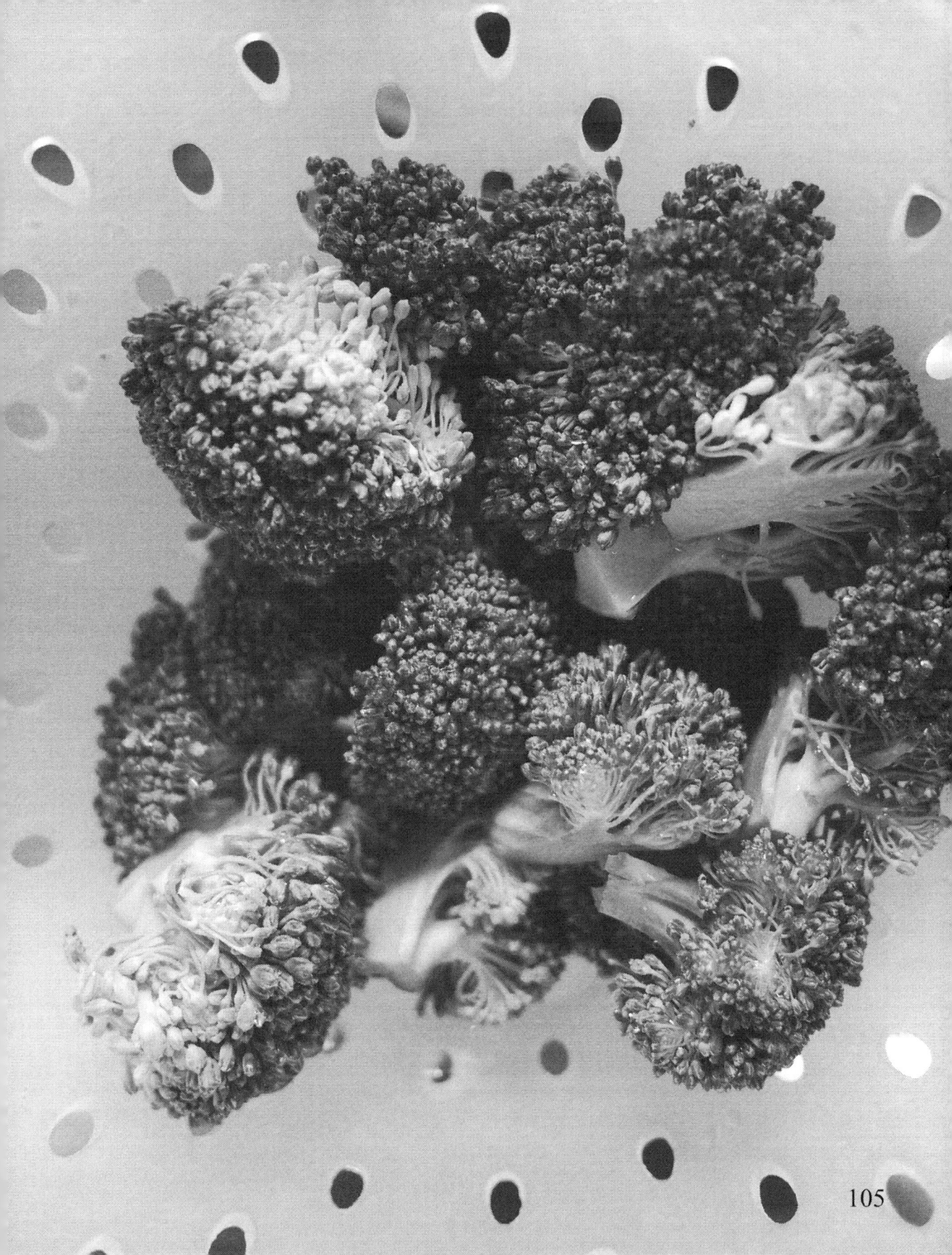

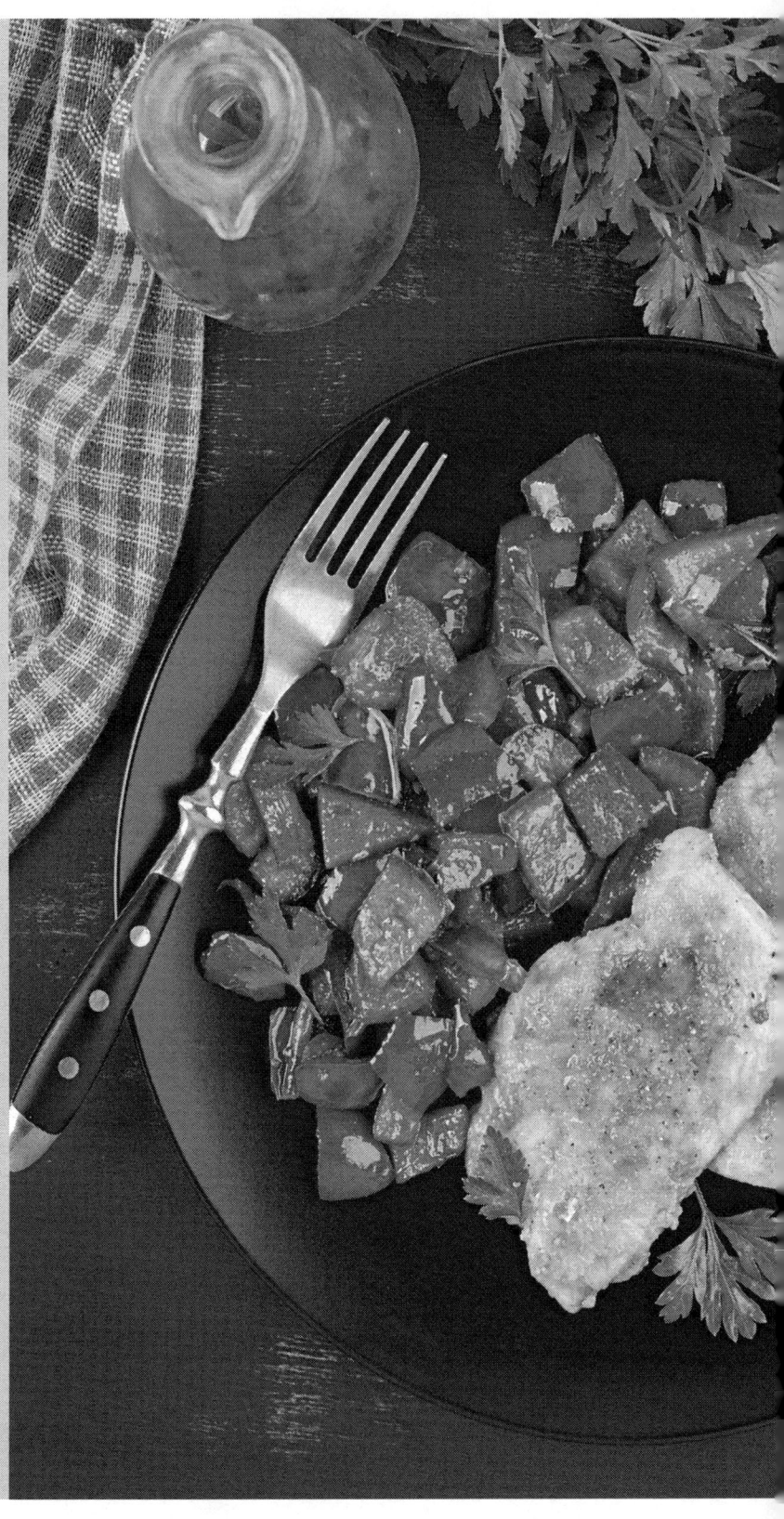

DINNER RECIPES

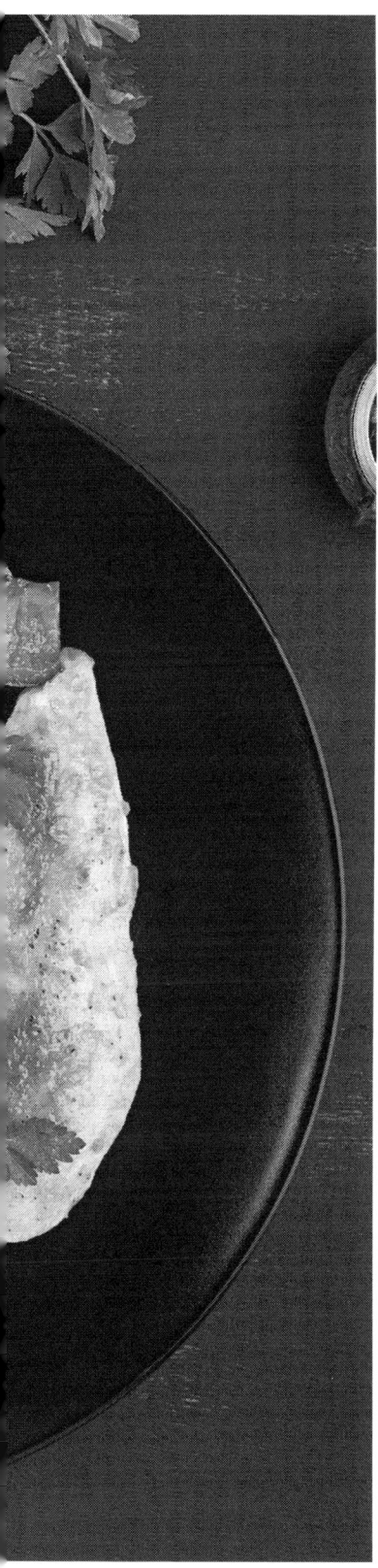

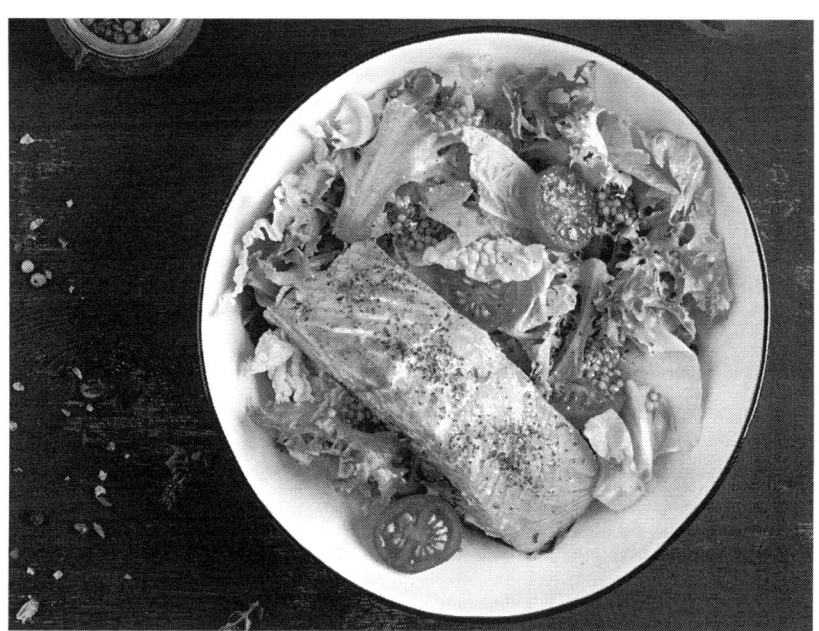

Recipes include foods recommended in the GOLO diet, such as lean sources of protein, lean dairy products, low glycemic index vegetables, whole grains, and healthy sources of fat. Recipes include low to medium GI ingredients to help maintain stable blood sugar levels.

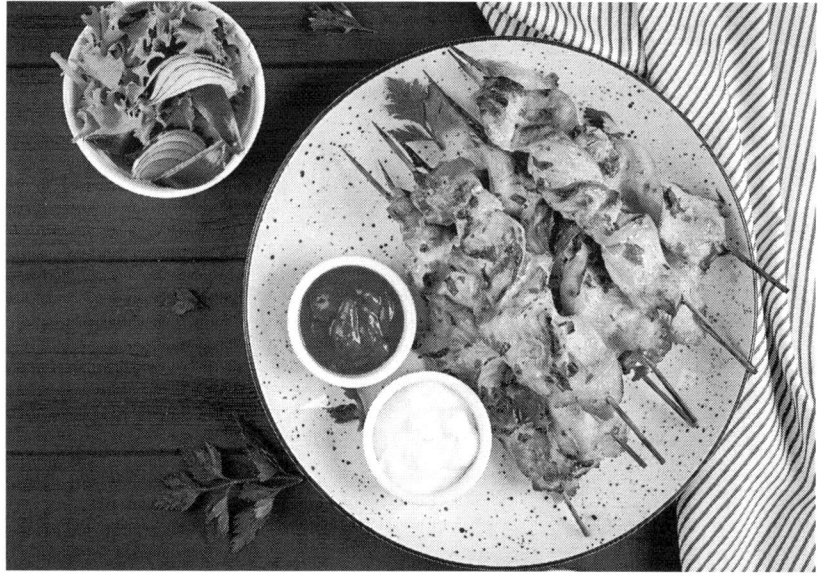

BAKED CHICKEN WITH SWEET PAPRIKA

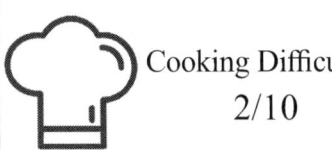 Cooking Difficulty: 2/10	 Cooking Time: 35 minutes	 Servings: 4

INGREDIENTS

- 4 chicken fillets
- 2 tbsp. sweet paprika
- 3 tbsp. olive oil
- 3 tbsp. dried garlic
- salt
- black pepper

DESCRIPTION

STEP 1
Preheat oven to 380 F.

STEP 2
Rub the chicken fillet with spices and olive oil and let sit for 5 minutes.

STEP 3
Place the chicken in the oven and bake for 30 minutes.

STEP 4
Serve with salad or chopped vegetables.

NUTRITIONAL INFORMATION

Calories 298, Fat 9,3g, Carbs 6g, Protein 11g

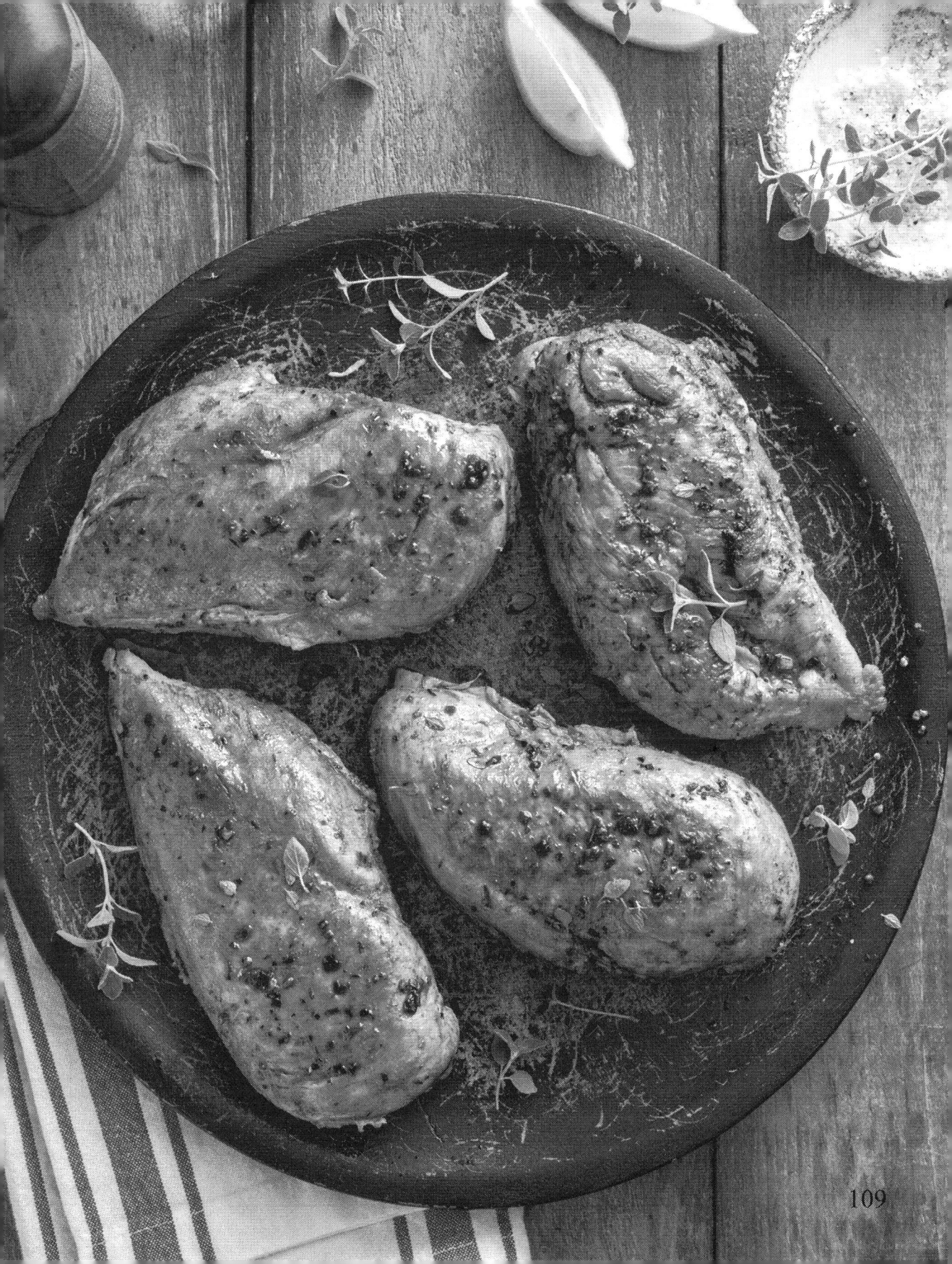

CHICKEN PIECES

 Cooking Difficulty: 3/10	 Cooking Time: 15 minutes	 Servings: 6

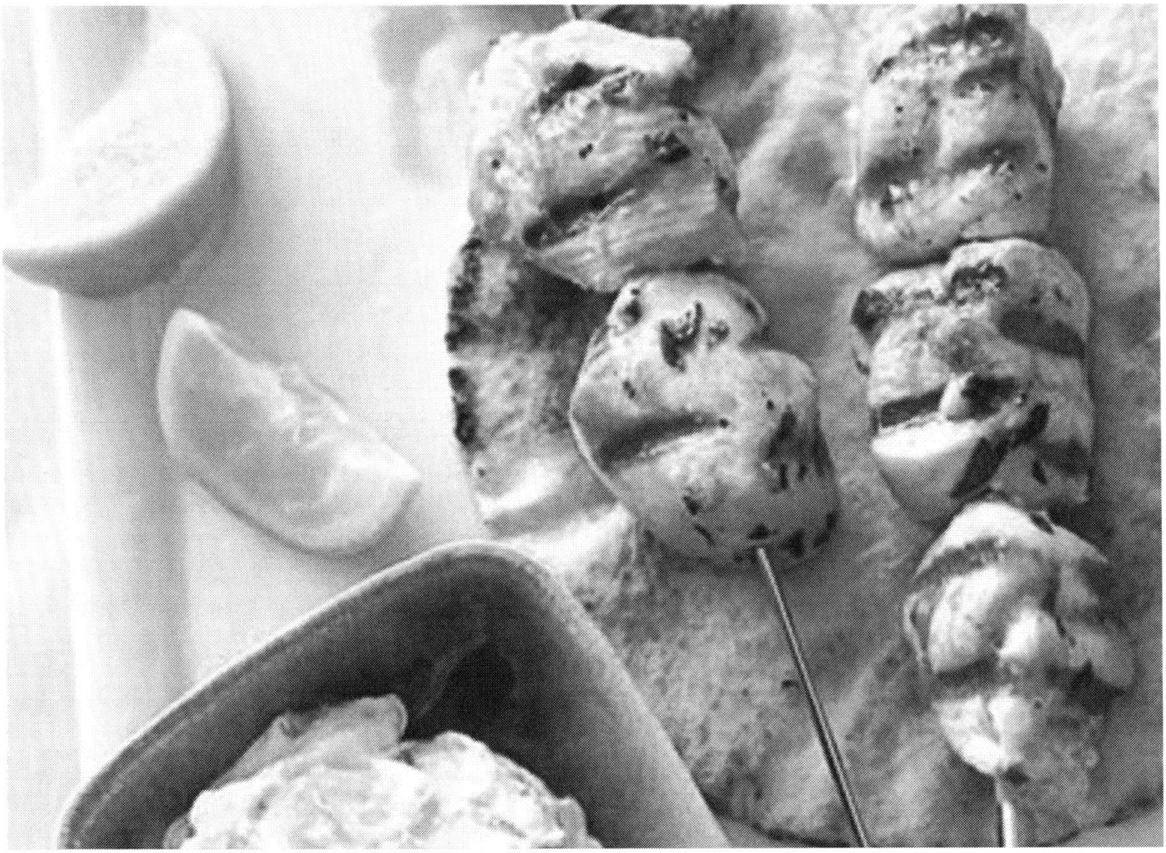

NUTRITIONAL INFORMATION

294 Calories, 5.2g Fat, 42.1g Carbs, 22.2g Protein

INGREDIENTS

- 2 tbsps. lemon juice
- 14 oz. greek yogurt
- 2 tsps. chopped oregano leaves
- ¼ c. white dry wine
- ¼ c. olive oil
- ½ tsp. pepper - divided
- 1 tsp. salt
- 2 lb. skinned breasts
- 4 minced garlic cloves
- 2 tsps. distilled white vinegar
- ½ c. cucumber

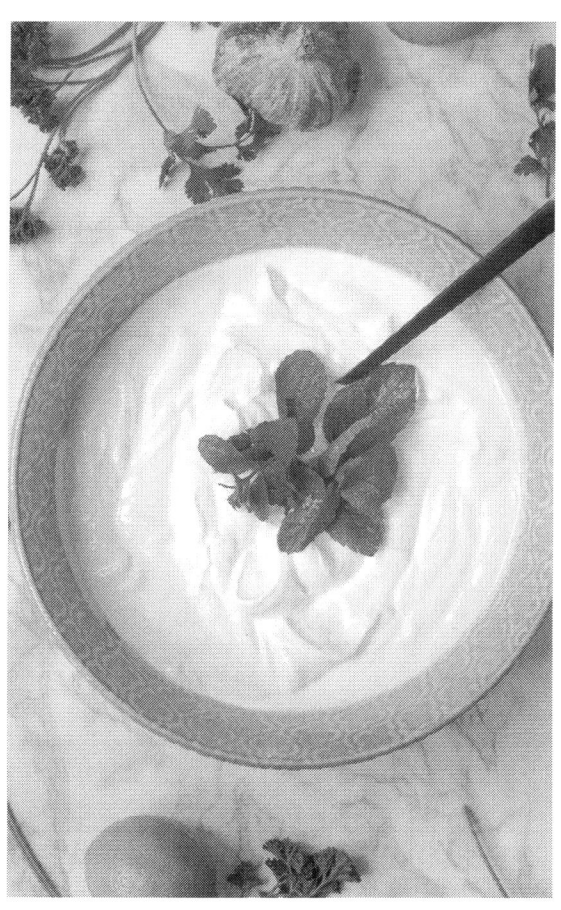

DESCRIPTION

STEP 1
Cut the chicken into ½-inch cubes, and coarsely shred the cucumber.

STEP 2
Set the grill between 450°F and 550°F.

STEP 3
Blend the wine, oil, chicken, oregano, lime juice, ¼ teaspoon of pepper, and salt in a mixing bowl.

STEP 4
Use eight metal skewers to prepare the chicken for cooking. Grill for approximately 10-12 minutes.

STEP 5
Remove any excess moisture from the cucumbers with paper towels, and put them into a medium dish. Mix in the yogurt, garlic, vinegar, and pepper with the cucumbers.

STEP 6
Serve with warm pita bread and chicken. Place remaining portions in an airtight container and refrigerate for up to 3 days.

111

SEA BASS

 Cooking Difficulty: 2/10

 Cooking Time: 18 minutes

 Servings: 2

INGREDIENTS

- 2 lemons
- 1/3 c. green olives
- 1 c. grated cauliflower
- 1 seabass
- pepper
- salt
- 1/3 c. chopped parsley
- 1/3 c. chopped mint

DESCRIPTION

STEP 1
Allow the oven to heat up to 400 degrees. Place some parchment paper on a baking pan and place the fish on top. Add some oil to the fish.

STEP 2
Slice the lemons and stuff them into the bass along with the herbs. Place into the oven to bake for 15 minutes.

STEP 3
Chop up the olives and juice the other lemons. Take out a bowl and mix together the rest of the ingredients.

STEP 4
Serve the prepared fish with the cauliflower salad.

NUTRITIONAL INFORMATION

380 Calories, 26g Fats, 3.4g Carbs, 11g Protein

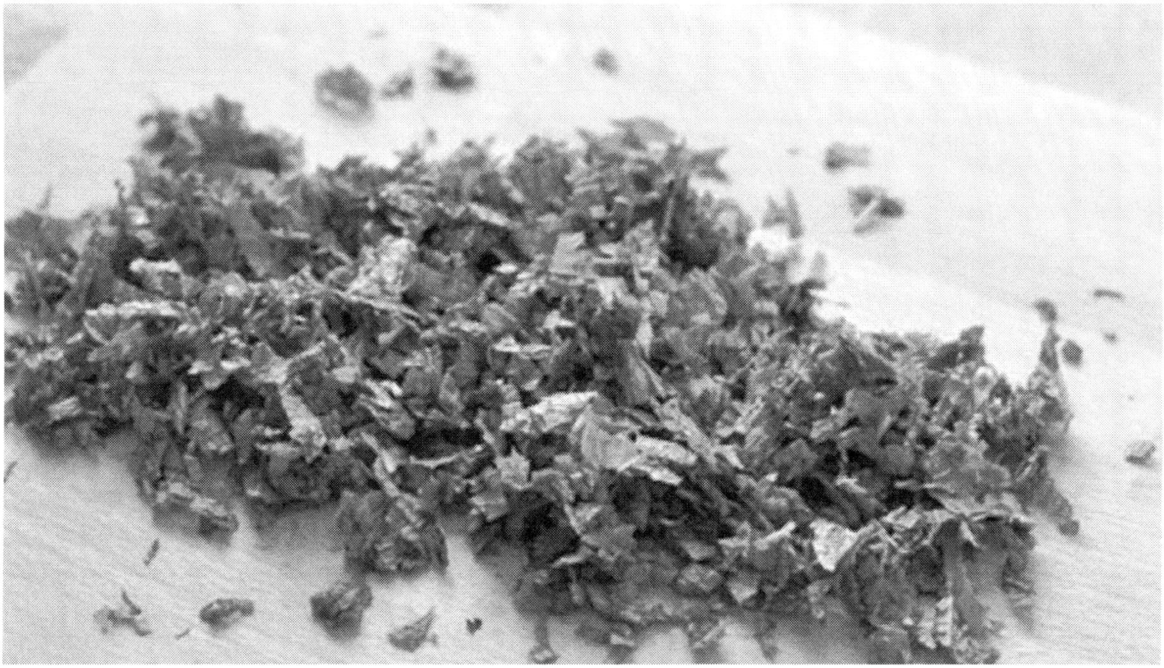

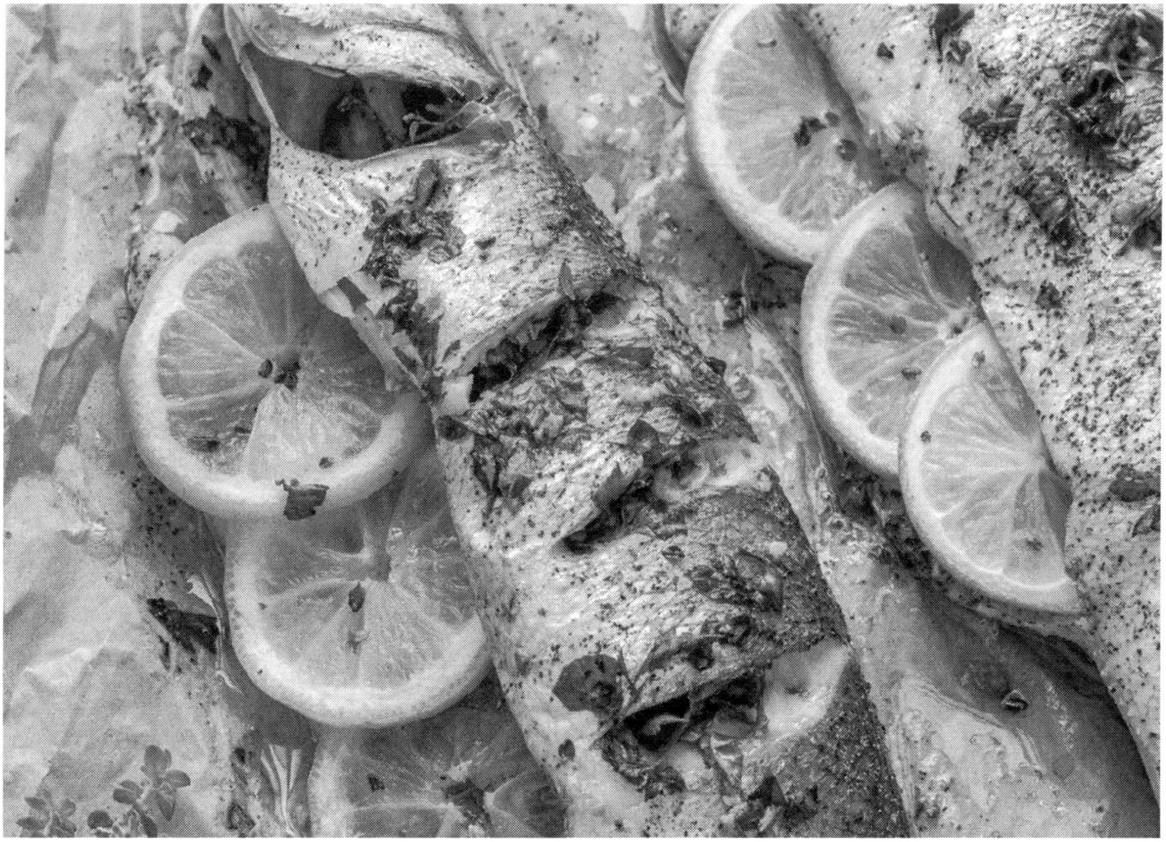

CUMIN SALMON

 Cooking Difficulty: 2/10	 Cooking Time: 7 minutes	 Servings: 4

INGREDIENTS

- 4 salmon fillets, boneless
- 1 tbsp. olive oil
- 1 sliced red onion
- salt
- black pepper
- 1 tsp. ground cumin

DESCRIPTION

STEP 1
Heat up a pan with the oil over medium-high heat, add the onion then cook for 2 minutes.

STEP 2
Add the fish, salt, pepper, and the cumin, cook for 4 minutes on each side, divide between plates and serve.

NUTRITIONAL INFORMATION

Calories 300, Fat 14g, Carbs 5g, Protein 20g

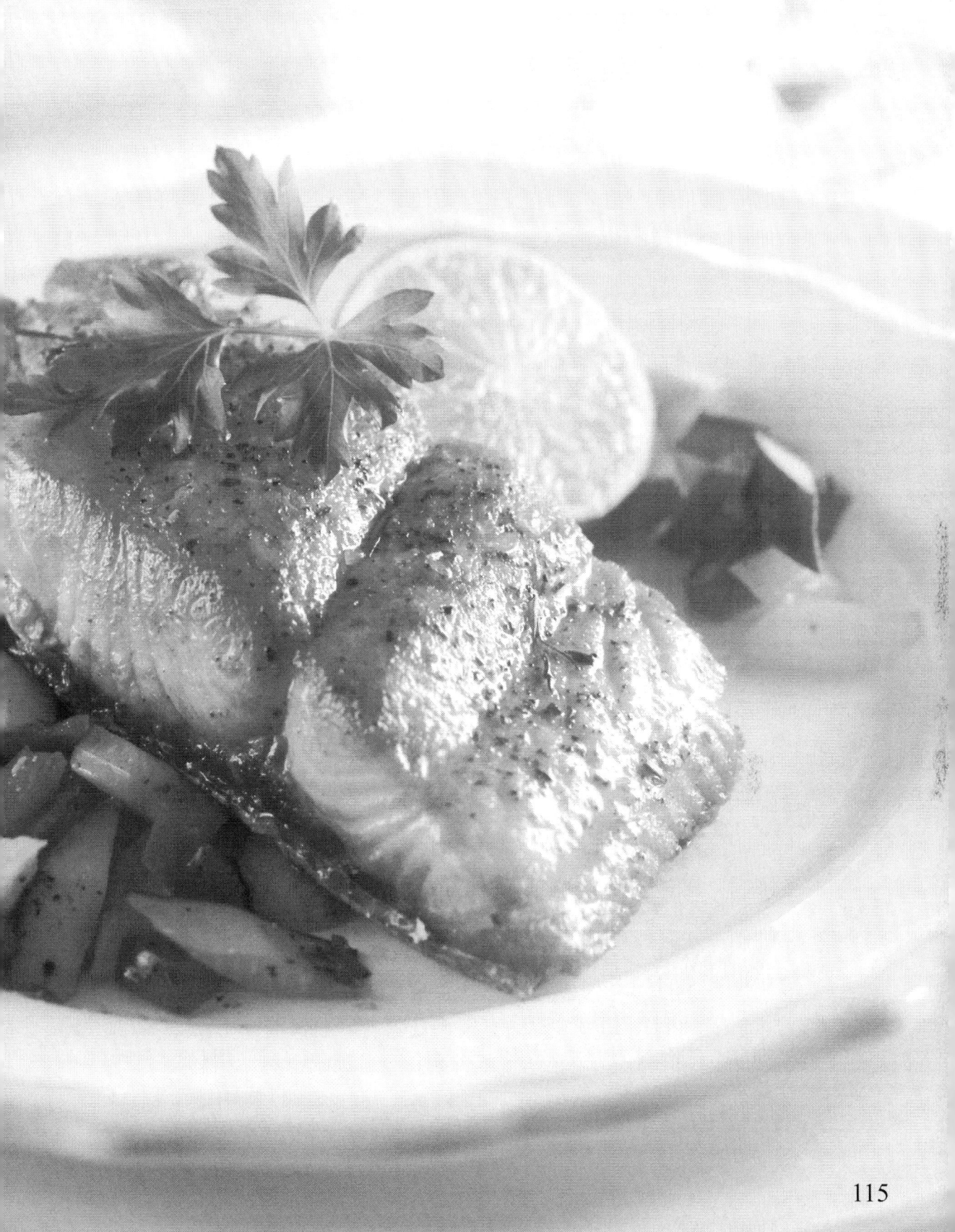

SHRIMP ZOODLES

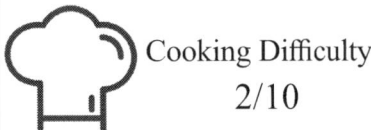 Cooking Difficulty: 2/10	 Cooking Time: 10 minutes	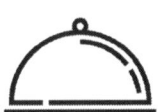 Servings: 4

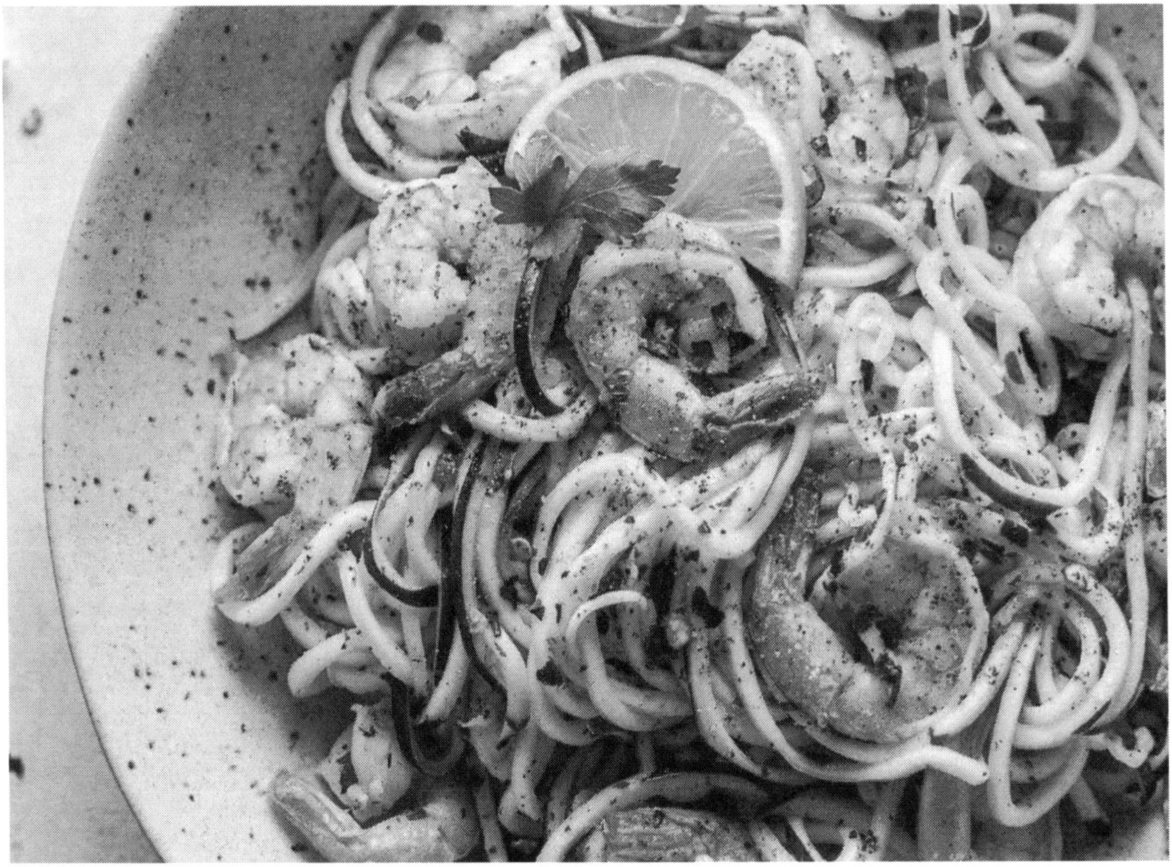

NUTRITIONAL INFORMATION

277 Calories, 15.6g Fat, 5.9g Carbs, 7.5g Protein

INGREDIENTS

- 4 c. zoodles
- 1 tbsp. chopped basil
- 1 lb. shrimp
- 1 c. vegetable stock
- 2 minced garlic cloves
- 2 tbsps. olive oil
- ½ lemon
- ½ tsp. paprika

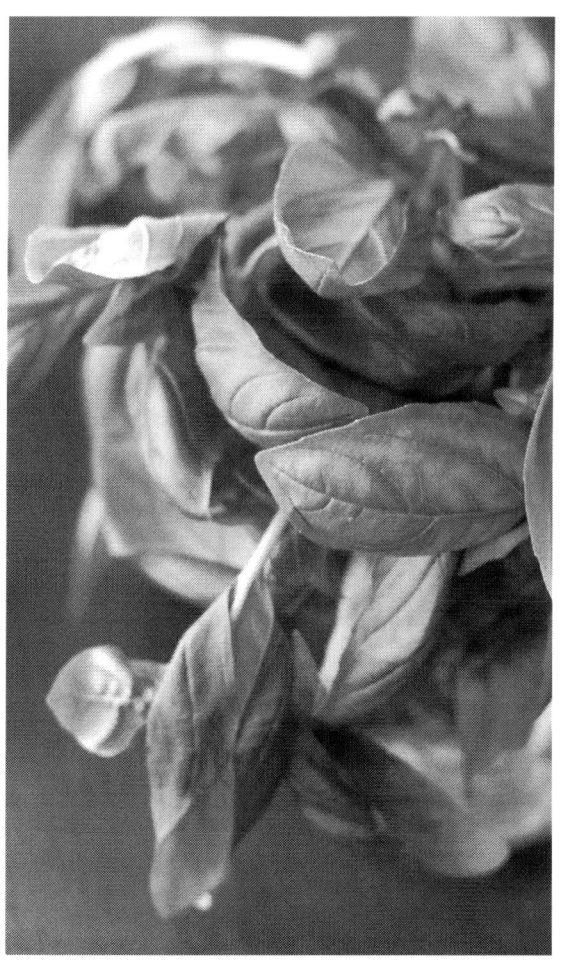

DESCRIPTION

STEP 1

Set your Instant Pot to SAUTÉ and add the olive oil in it.

STEP 2

Add garlic and cook for 1 minute.

STEP 3

Add the lemon juice and shrimp and cook for another minute.

STEP 4

Stir in the remaining ingredients and close the lid.

STEP 5

Set the Instant Pot to MANUAL and cook at low pressure for 5 minutes.

STEP 6

Do a quick pressure release.

STEP 7

Serve and enjoy!

DELICIOUS SALMON

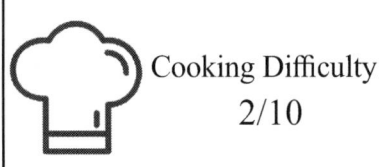 Cooking Difficulty: 2/10	 Cooking Time: 16 minutes	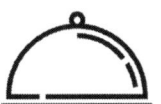 Servings: 2

INGREDIENTS

- 2 salmon steak
- 1 tbsp. olive oil
- salt
- pepper
- half a lemon
- salad leaves for serving

DESCRIPTION

STEP 1
Heat up a pan with the oil over medium-high heat.

STEP 2
Add fish, salt, and pepper, cook for 4 minutes on each side, divide onto plates and serve with your favorite salad and lemon.

NUTRITIONAL INFORMATION

362 Calories, 7g Fats, 4.7g Carbs, 5.8 Protein

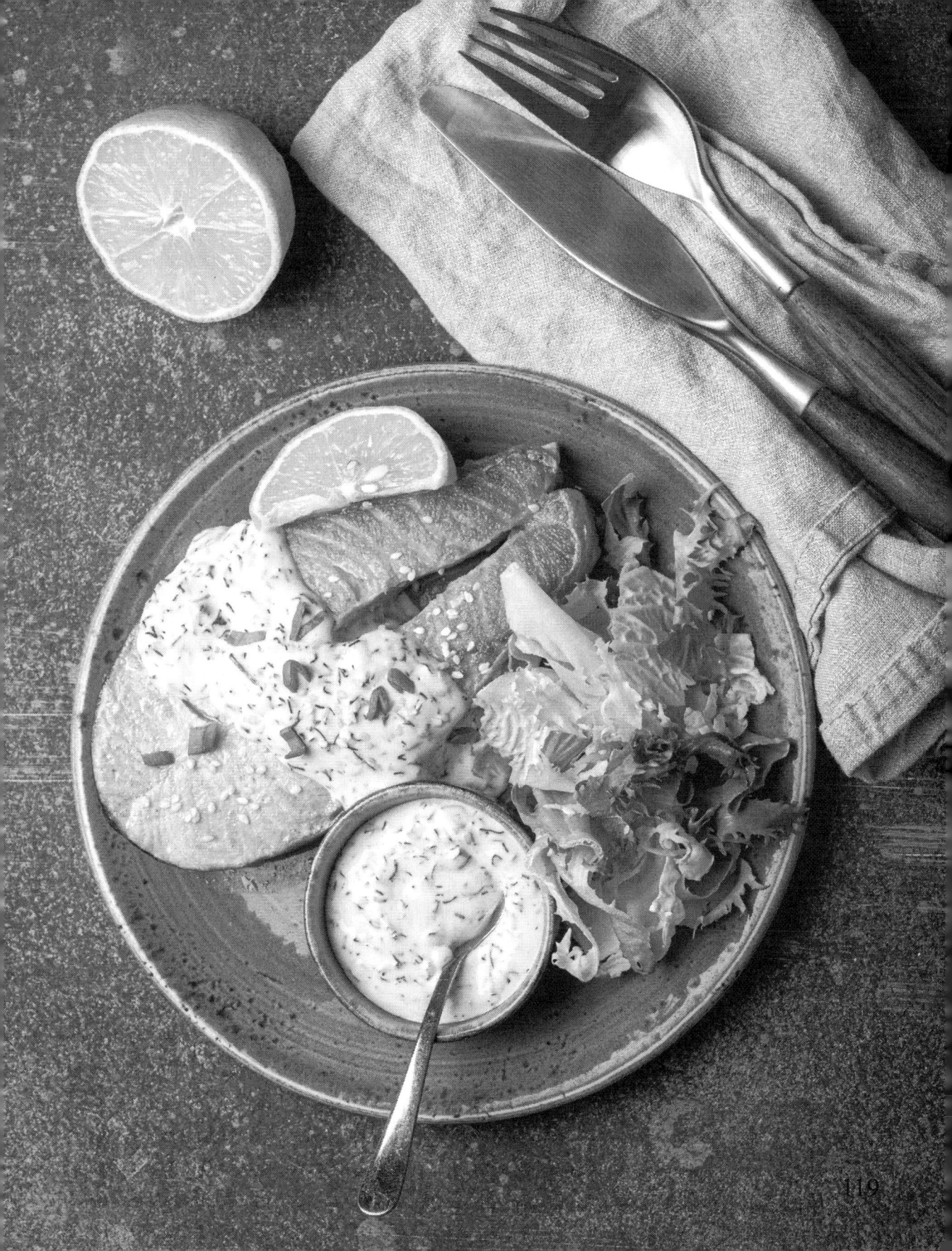

CAULIFLOWER BOLOGNESE WITH ZUCCHINI NOODLES

 Cooking Difficulty: 2/10

 Cooking Time: 8 minutes

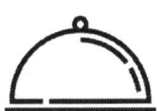 Servings: 2

INGREDIENTS

- 1 medium head cauliflower, broken into florets
- 2 minced cloves garlic
- ½ c. diced onions
- ¾ tsp. dried basil
- red pepper flakes
- 1 tsp. dried oregano flakes
- ¼ c. chicken broth
- 1½ cans (14 oz. each) diced tomatoes
- 3 zucchinis

DESCRIPTION

STEP 1
Add all the ingredients except zucchini to the Instant Pot. Close the lid. Select MANUAL and cook at high pressure for 3 minutes. When the cooking is complete, do a quick pressure release.

STEP 2
Meanwhile, make noodles of the zucchini using a spiralizer using blade A or a julienne peeler. Mash the cauliflower with a potato masher or in a food processor.

STEP 3
Divide the noodles in 2 bowls. Place cauliflower Bolognese over it and serve.

NUTRITIONAL INFORMATION

Calories: 210; Fat: 1.9 g; Carbs: 28.1; Protein: 14.3 g

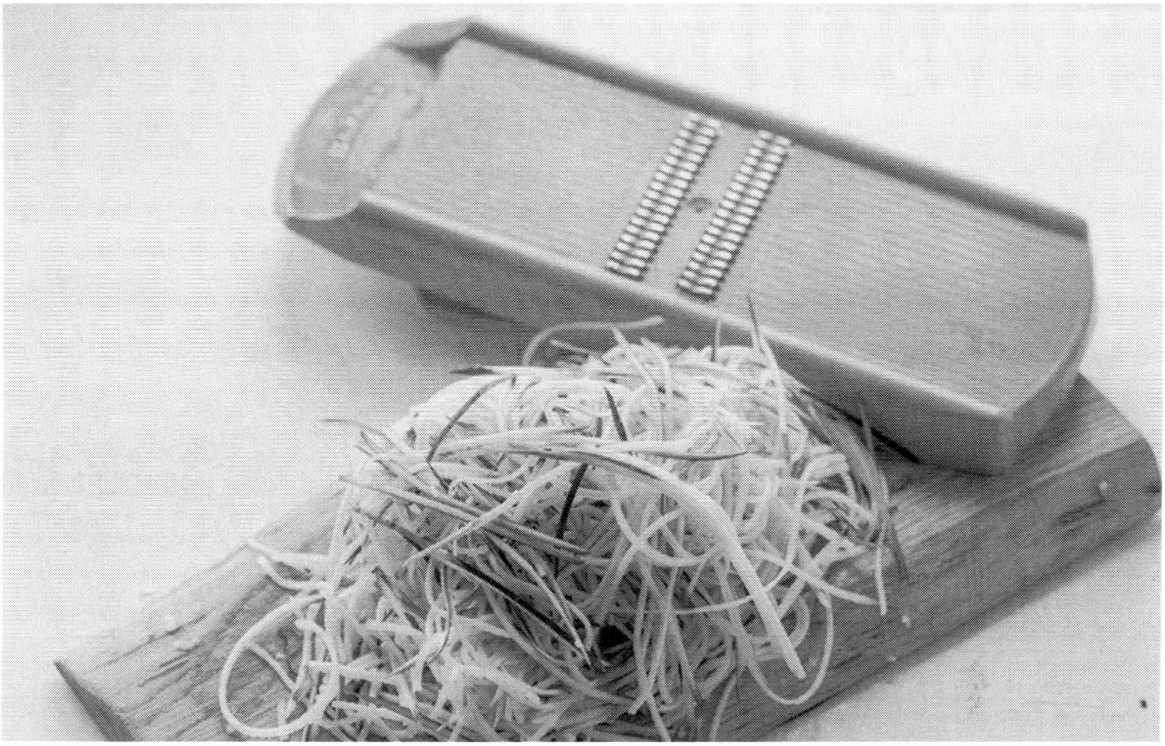

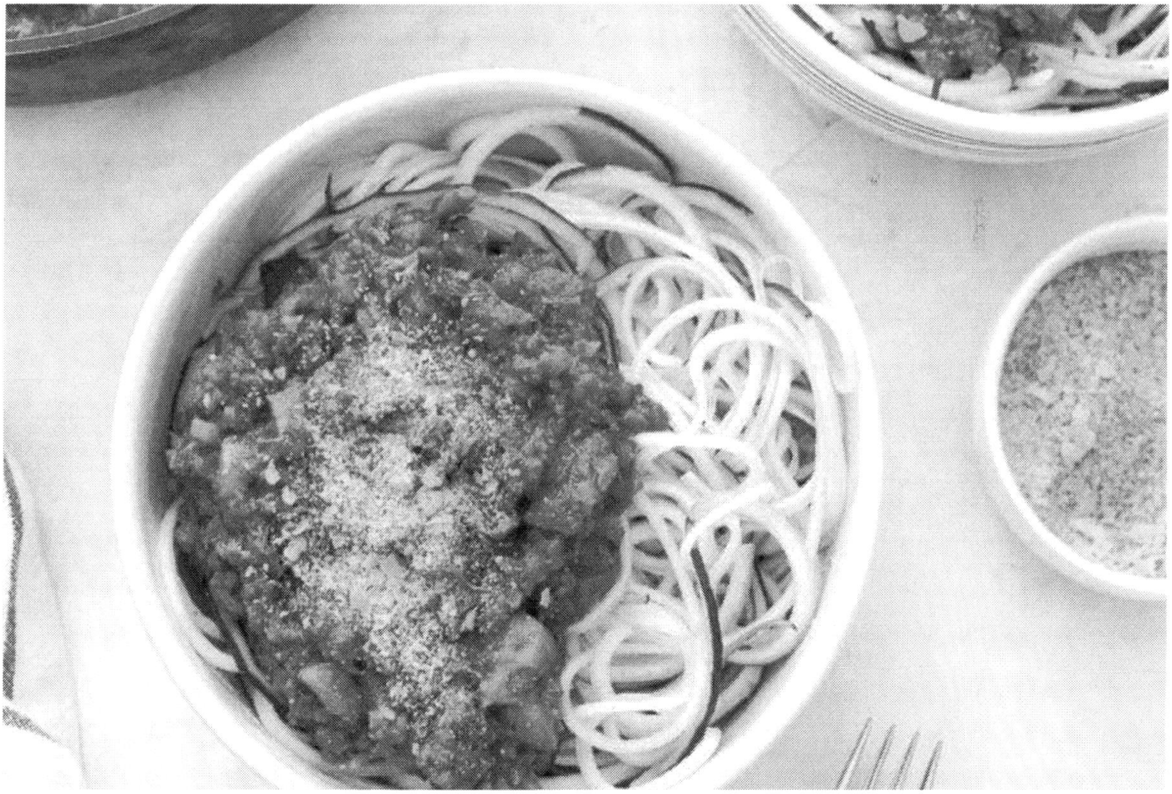

CHICKPEA AND SPINACH CUTLETS

 Cooking Difficulty: 3/10	 Cooking Time: 40 minutes	 Servings: 12

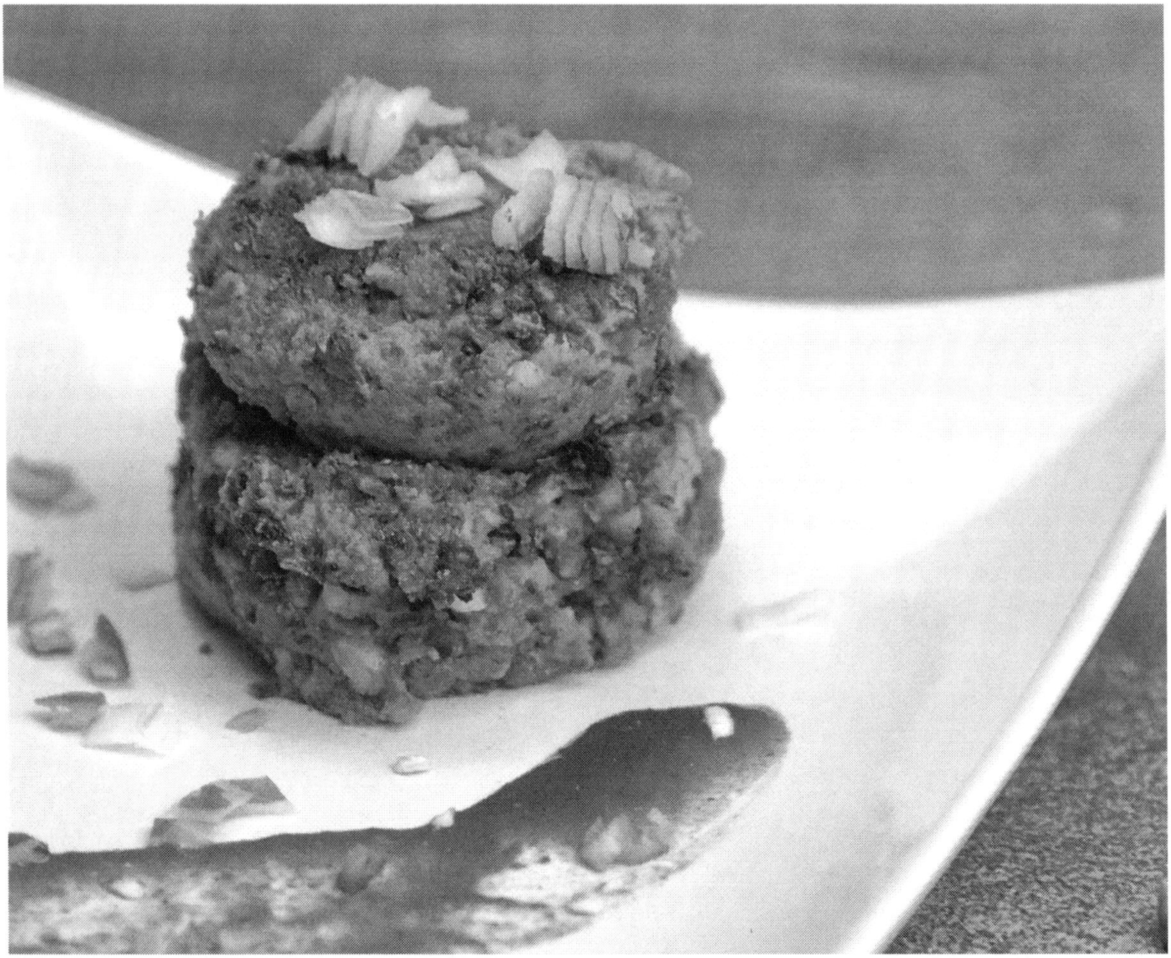

NUTRITIONAL INFORMATION

170 Calories, 5g Fat, 1.7g Carbs, 4g Protein

INGREDIENTS

- 1 red bell pepper
- 19 oz. chickpeas, rinsed & drained
- 1 c. ground almonds
- 2 tsps. dijon mustard
- 1 tsp. oregano
- 1 c. spinach, fresh
- 1½ c. rolled oats
- 1 clove garlic, pressed
- ½ lemon, juiced

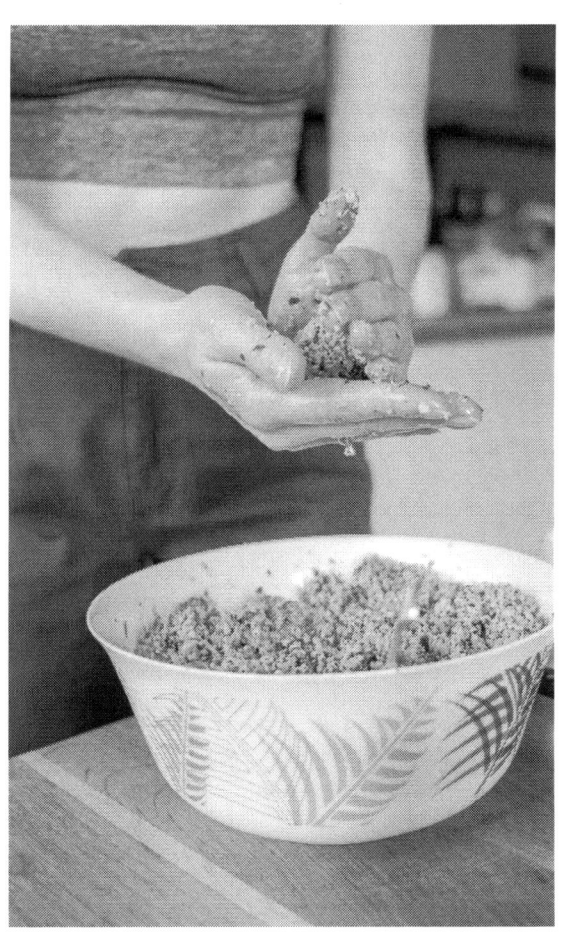

DESCRIPTION

STEP 1
Get out a baking sheet. Line it with parchment paper.

STEP 2
Cut your red pepper in half and then take the seeds out. Place it on your baking sheet, and roast it in the oven while you prepare your other ingredients.

STEP 3
Process your chickpeas, almonds, and mustard together in a food processor.

STEP 4
Add in your lemon juice, oregano, sage, garlic, and spinach, processing again. Make sure it's combined, but don't puree it.

STEP 5
Once your red bell pepper is softened, which should roughly take ten minutes, add this to the processor as well. Add in your oats, mixing well.

STEP 6
Form twelve patties, cooking in the oven for a half hour. They should be browned.

SPINACH WITH GARBANZO BEANS

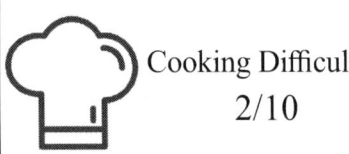 Cooking Difficulty: 2/10

 Cooking Time: 8 minutes

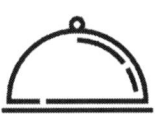 Servings: 4

INGREDIENTS

- 1 tbsp. olive oil
- 4 minced garlic cloves
- ½ diced onion
- 10 oz. chopped spinach
- 12 oz. garbanzo beans
- ½ tsp. cumin
- ½ tsp. salt

DESCRIPTION

STEP 1
In a skillet, warm the olive oil over medium-low heat.

STEP 2
Then add the onions and garlic and cook until the onions are translucent. About 5 minutes.

STEP 3
Stir in spinach, cumin, salt, and garbanzo beans.

STEP 4
Allow cooking until thoroughly heated.

NUTRITIONAL INFORMATION

90 Calories, 4g Fat, 11g Carbs, 4g Protein

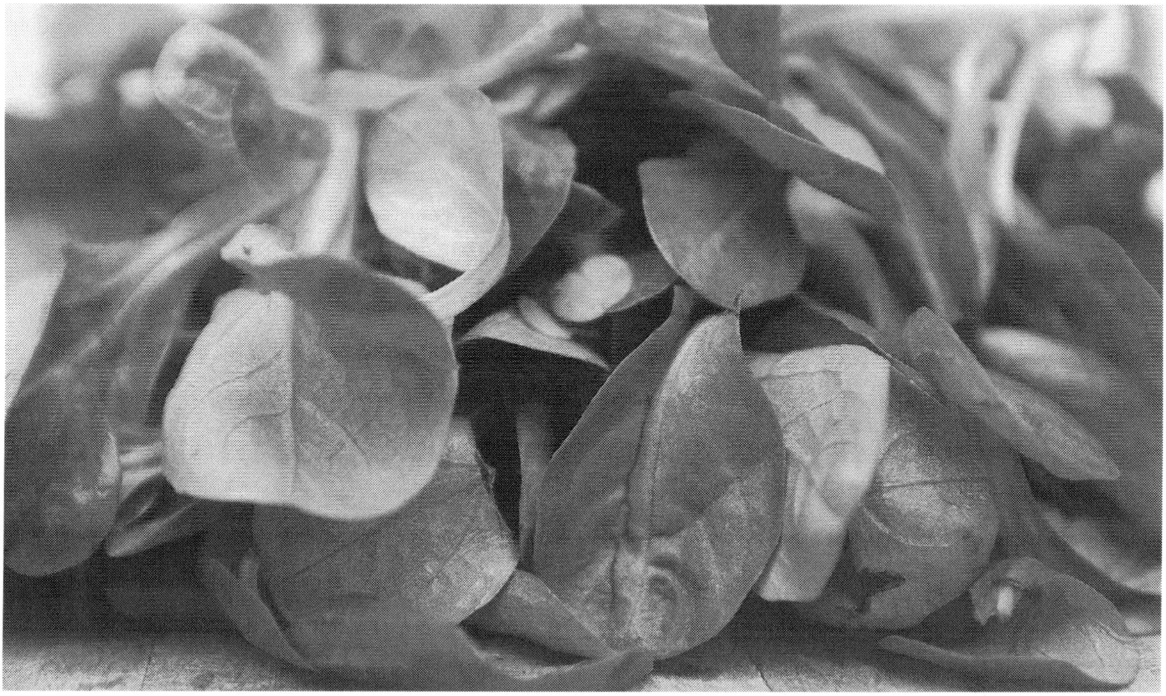

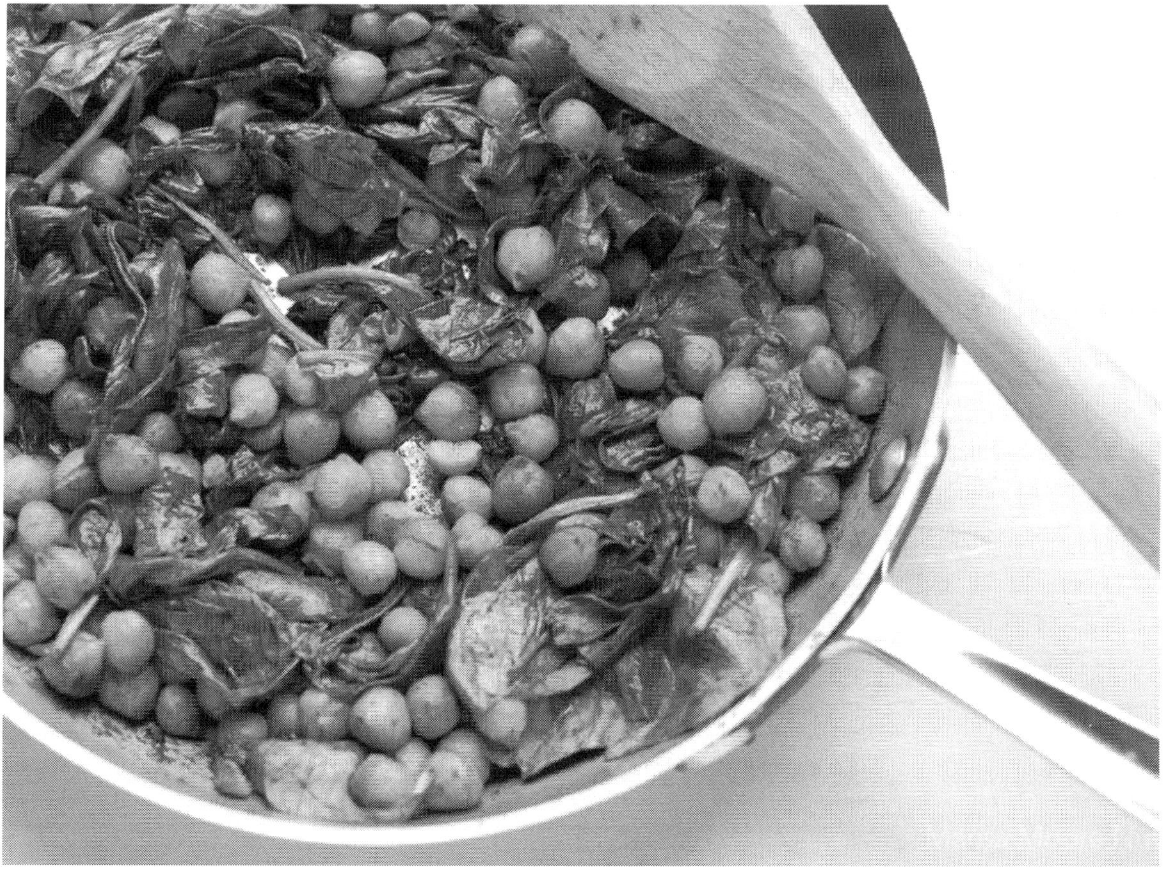

CHIVES TROUT

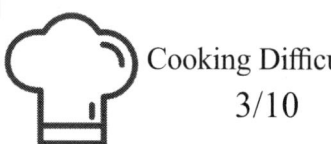 Cooking Difficulty: 3/10

 Cooking Time: 7 minutes

 Servings: 4

INGREDIENTS

- 4 boneless trout fillets
- 2 shallots, chopped
- salt
- black pepper
- 3 tbsps. chopped chives
- 2 tbsps. olive oil
- 2 tsps. lime juice

DESCRIPTION

STEP 1
Ensure that you heat the pan, add the shallots, and sauté them for 2 minutes.

STEP 2
Add the fish, and the rest of the ingredients cook for 5 minutes on each side, divide between plate and serve. Place remaining portions in an airtight container and refrigerate for up to 2 days.

NUTRITIONAL INFORMATION

Calories 320, Fat 12g, Carbs 2g, Protein 24g

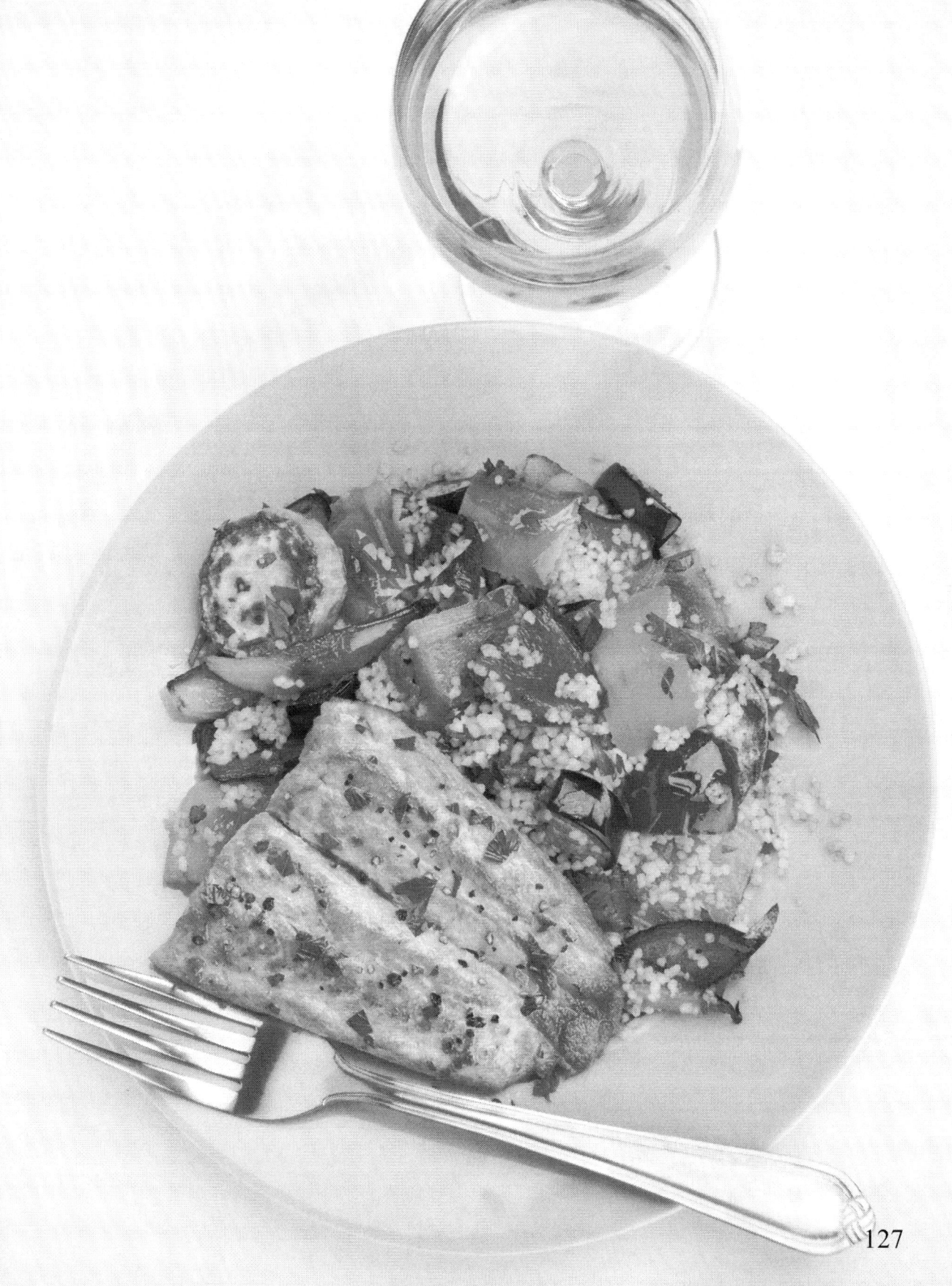

CAULIFLOWER STEAK WITH SWEET-PEA PUREE

 Cooking Difficulty: 3/10	 Cooking Time: 35 minutes	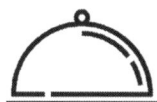 Servings: 2

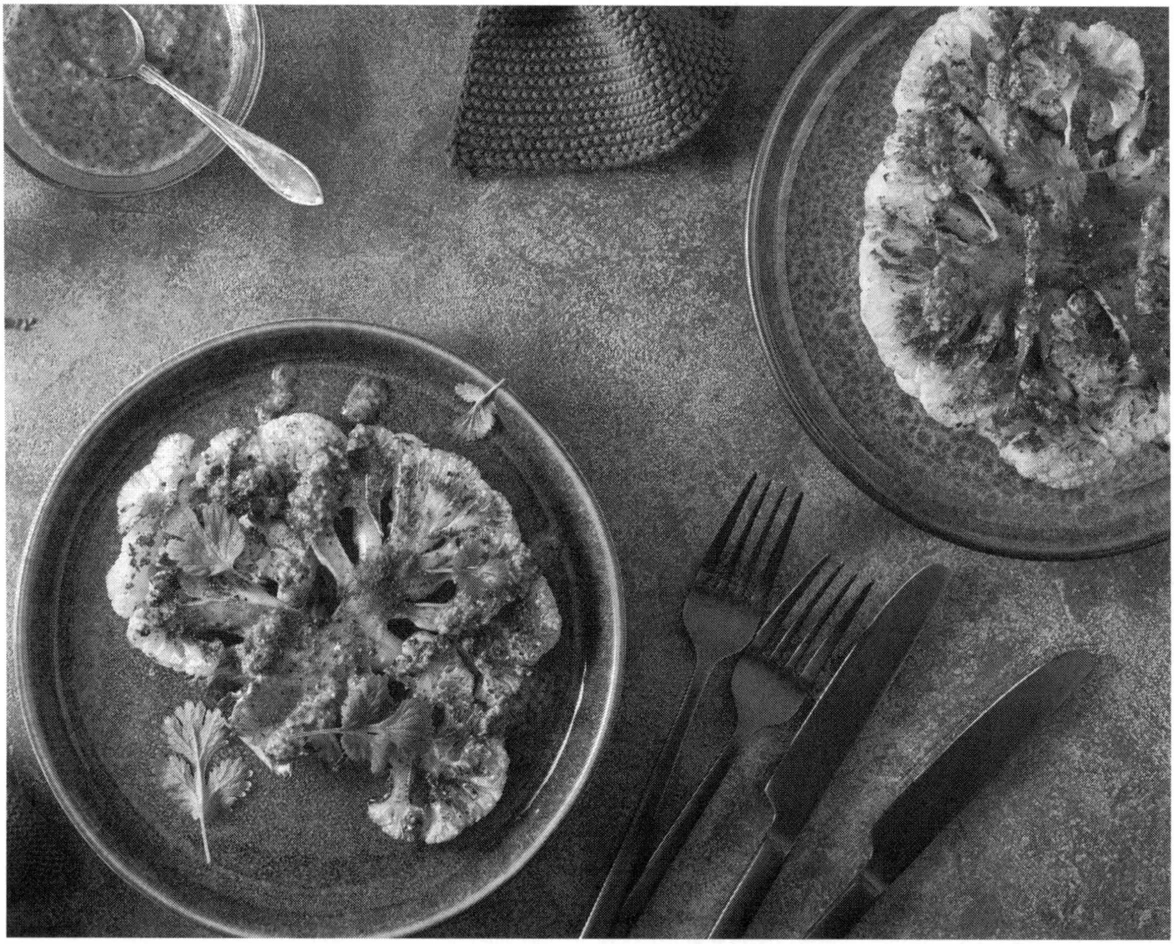

NUTRITIONAL INFORMATION

Calories 234, Fat 3.8g, Carbs 40.3g, Protein 14.5g

INGREDIENTS

cauliflower:
- 2 heads cauliflower
- 1 tsp. olive oil
- ¼ tsp. paprika
- ¼ tsp. black pepper

sweet-pea puree:
- 10 oz. frozen green peas
- 1 onion, chopped
- 2 tbsps. fresh parsley
- ¼ c. unsweetened vegan milk

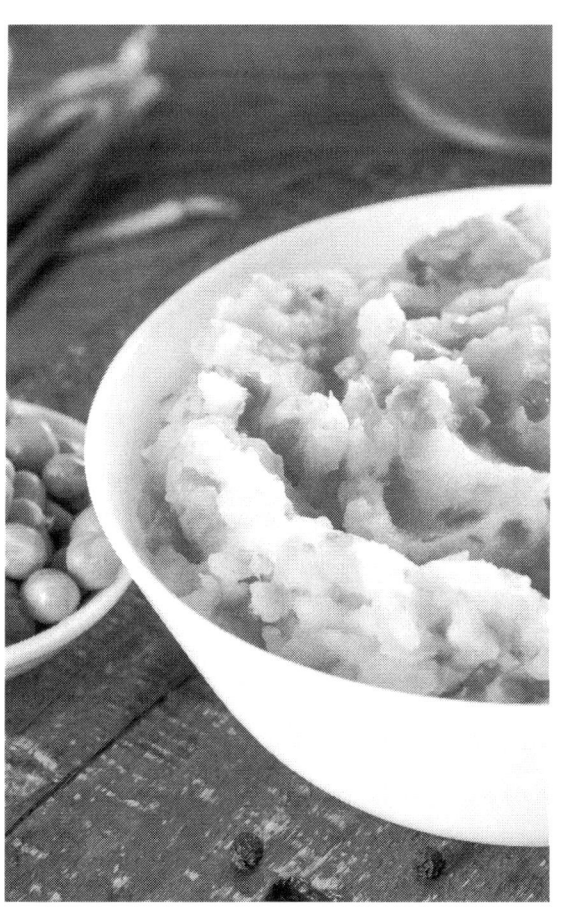

DESCRIPTION

STEP 1
Preheat oven to 425F.

STEP 2
Remove bottom core of cauliflower. Stand it on its base, starting in the middle, slice in half. Then slice steaks about ¾ inches thick.

STEP 3
Using a baking pan, set in the steaks.

STEP 4
Using olive oil, coat the front and back of the steaks.

STEP 5
Sprinkle with paprika, and pepper.

STEP 6
Bake for 30 minutes, flipping once.

STEP 7
Meanwhile, steam the chopped onion and peas until soft.

STEP 8
Place these vegetables in a blender with milk and parsley and blend until smooth.

GINGER HALIBUT

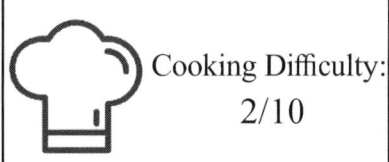 Cooking Difficulty: 2/10

 Cooking Time: 18 minutes

 Servings: 3

INGREDIENTS

- 24 oz. Alaskan halibut fillets
- 1½ tbsps. minced fresh ginger
- 1½ tsps. soy sauce
- 1½ tsps. olive oil
- ¾ tsp. rice wine vinegar

DESCRIPTION

STEP 1
Set the oven to 400 degrees F to preheat. Line a baking sheet with aluminum foil and set it aside.

STEP 2
Combine rice vinegar and olive oils in a bowl, then stir in the soy sauce, and ginger. Add the fish fillets and turn several times to coat.

STEP 3
Arrange the fish fillets on the prepared baking sheet—Bake for 17 minutes, or until done

NUTRITIONAL INFORMATION

380 Calories, 6g Fats, 3.4g Carbs, 7g Protein

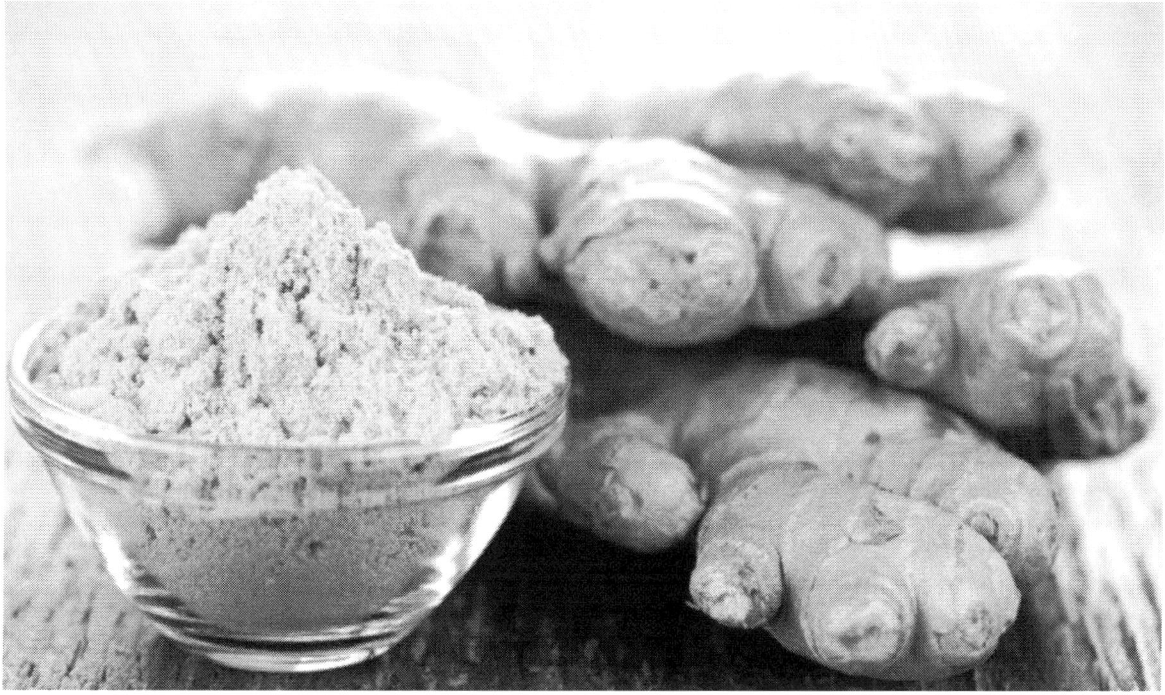

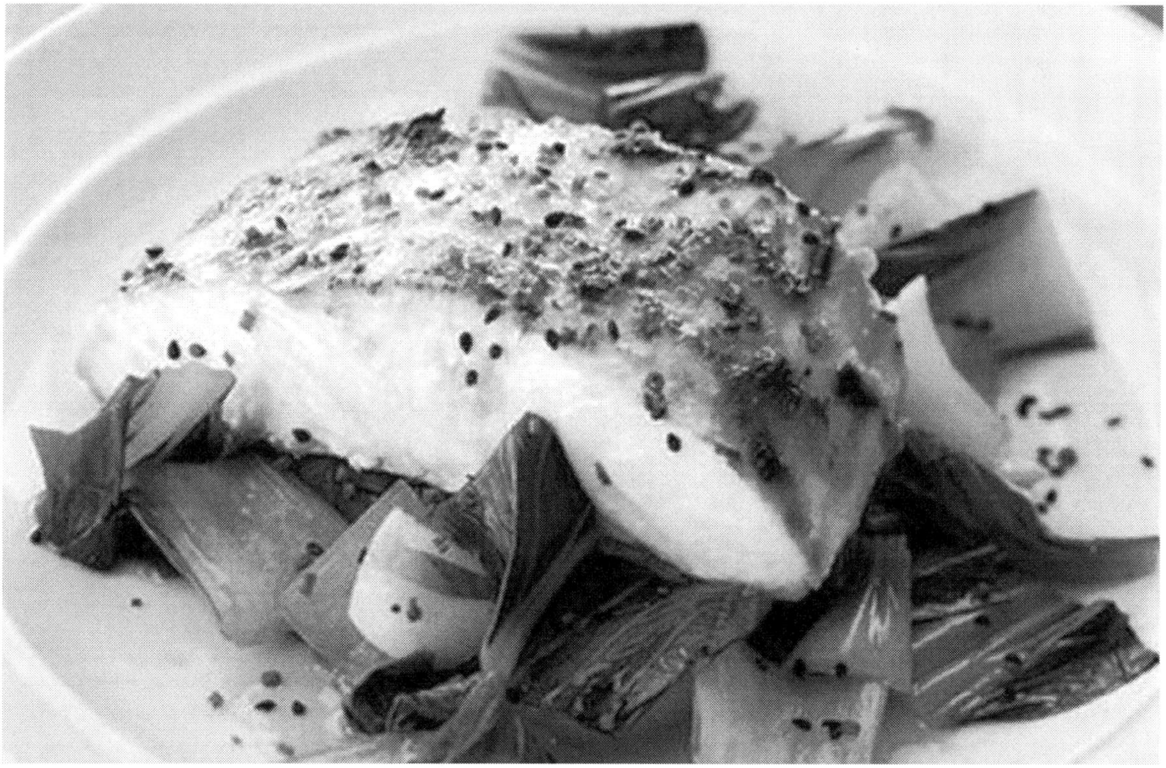

TOMATO TURKEY MEATBALLS

 Cooking Difficulty: 2/10

 Cooking Time: 11 minutes

 Servings: 4

INGREDIENTS

- ground turkey, 1 lb.
- diced onion, ¼
- almond flour, 1/3 c.
- garlic powder, ½ tsp.
- chicken stock, ¼ c.
- diced tomatoes, 28 oz.
- olive oil, 1 tbsp.
- basil, ½ tsp.
- pepper, ¼ tsp.

DESCRIPTION

STEP 1
In a bowl, mix the turkey, onion, almond flour until well combined.

STEP 2
Shape the mixture into small meatballs. Place the remaining ingredients in your Instant Pot and stir to combine.

STEP 3
Place the meatballs inside. Close the lid and set the Instant Pot to MANUAL. Cook on HIGH for 10 minutes.

STEP 4
Release the pressure quickly. Serve and enjoy!

NUTRITIONAL INFORMATION

350 Calories, 20.6g Fats, 6.9g Carbs, 38g Protein

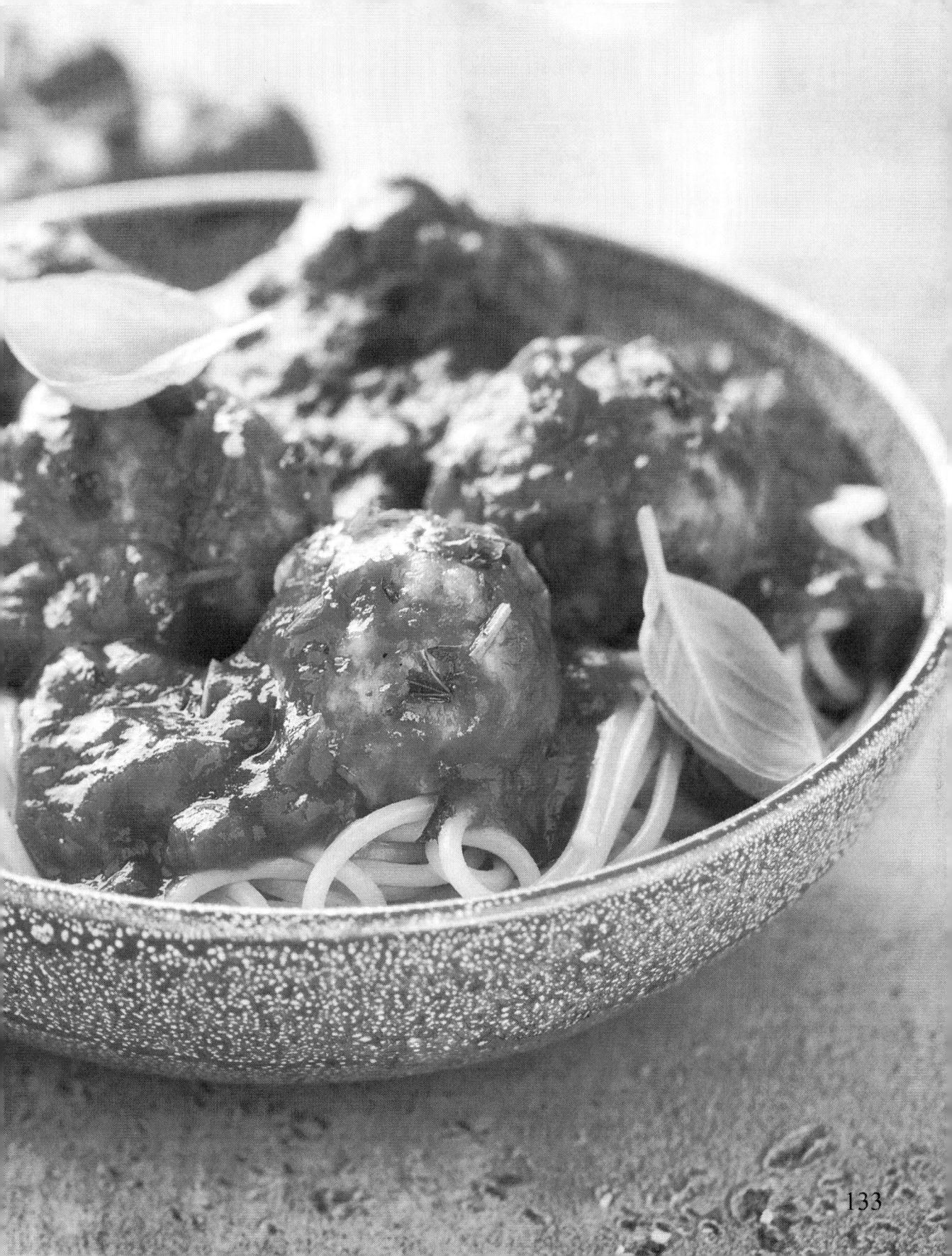

SWEET POTATO AND WHITE BEAN SKILLET

 Cooking Difficulty: 4/10	 Cooking Time: 30 minutes	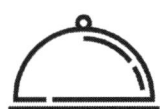 Servings: 4

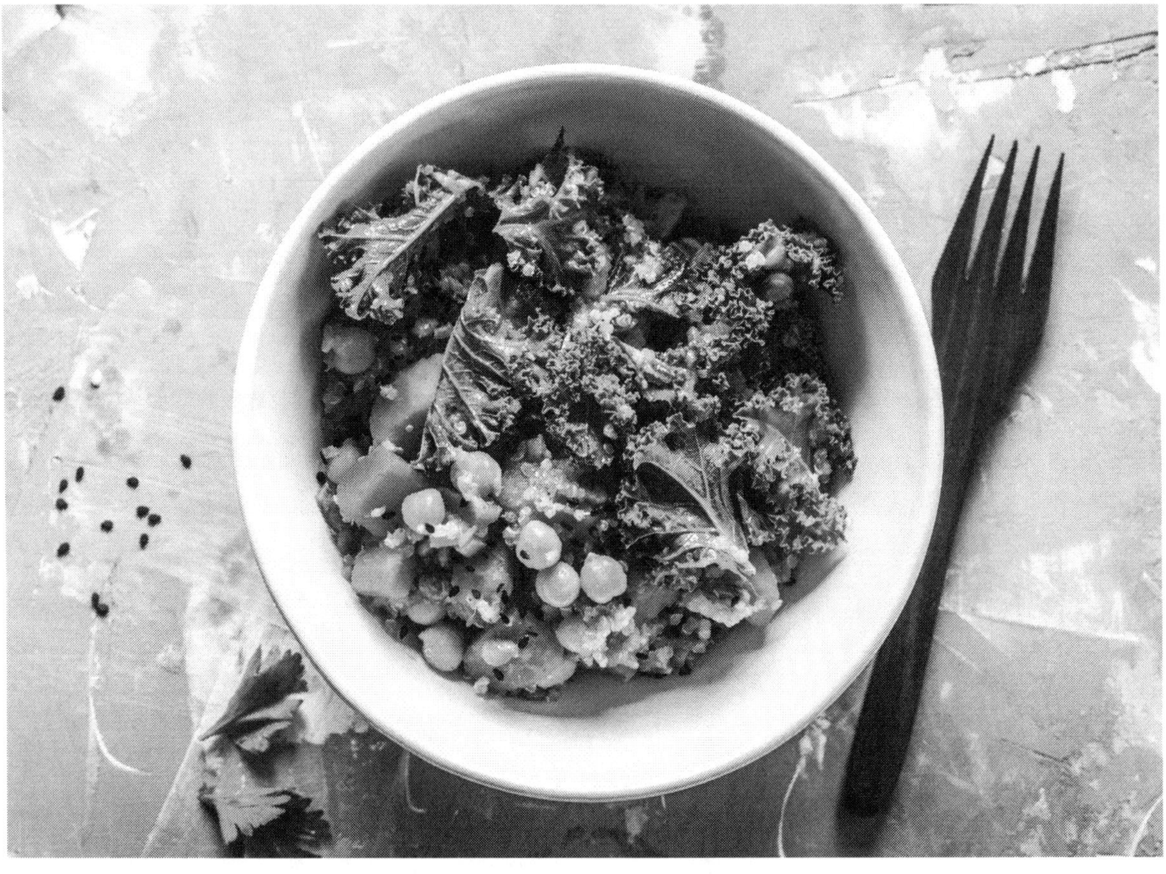

NUTRITIONAL INFORMATION

Calories: 260, Fat: 4 g, Carbs: 44 g, Protein: 13 g

INGREDIENTS

- 1 bunch kale, chopped
- 2 sweet potatoes, peeled, cubed
- 12 oz. cannellini beans
- 1 peeled onion, diced
- 1/8 tsp. red pepper flakes
- 1 tsp. salt
- ½ tsp. black pepper
- 1 tsp. curry powder
- 1 ½ tbsps. coconut oil
- 6 oz. coconut milk
- chickpeas (optional)

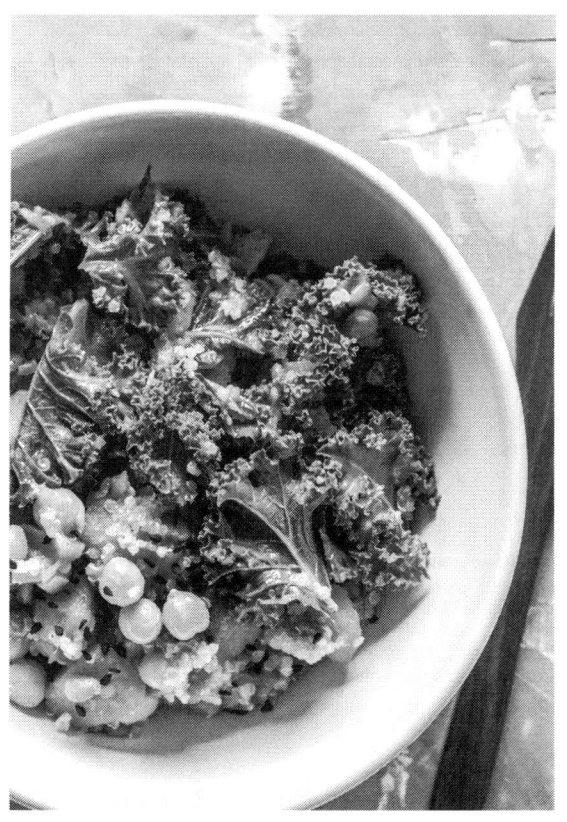

DESCRIPTION

STEP 1
Take a large skillet pan, place it over medium heat, add ½ tablespoon oil and when it melts, add onion and cook for 5 minutes.

STEP 2
Then stir in sweet potatoes, stir well, cook for 5 minutes, then season with all the spices, cook for 1 minute and remove the pan from heat.

STEP 3
Take another pan, add remaining oil in it, place it over medium heat and when oil melts, add kale, season with some salt and black pepper, stir well, pour in the milk and cook for 15 minutes until tender.

STEP 4
Then add beans, beans, and red pepper, stir until mixed and cook for 5 minutes until hot.

STEP 5
Serve straight away.

CABBAGE AND CHICKEN MIX

 Cooking Difficulty: 3/10

 Cooking Time: 22 minutes

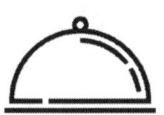 Servings: 4

INGREDIENTS

- ¼ tsp. red pepper, crushed
- ¼ c. chicken stock
- ¾ c. red bell peppers, chopped
- 3 tomatoes, cubed
- ¼ c. green onions, chopped
- 1 yellow onion, chopped
- 1 lb. chicken ground
- 1 green cabbage head, shredded
- 1 tbsp. olive oil
- salt
- pepper

DESCRIPTION

STEP 1

Heat up a pan with the oil over medium heat, add the chicken and the onions, stir and brown for 5 minutes.

STEP 2

Add the cabbage and the other ingredients, toss, cook for 15 minutes, divide into bowls and serve for lunch.

STEP 2

Place remaining portions in an airtight container and refrigerate for up to 3 days.

NUTRITIONAL INFORMATION

340 Calories, 10g Fats, 4g Carbs, 4.9 Protein

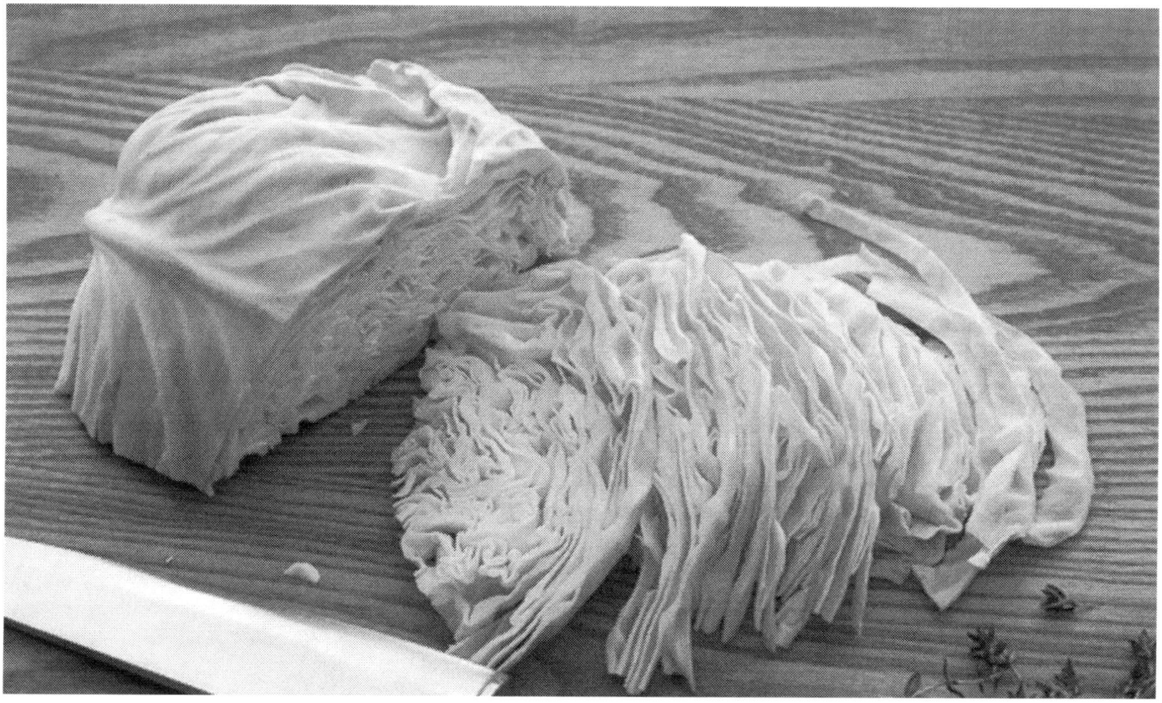

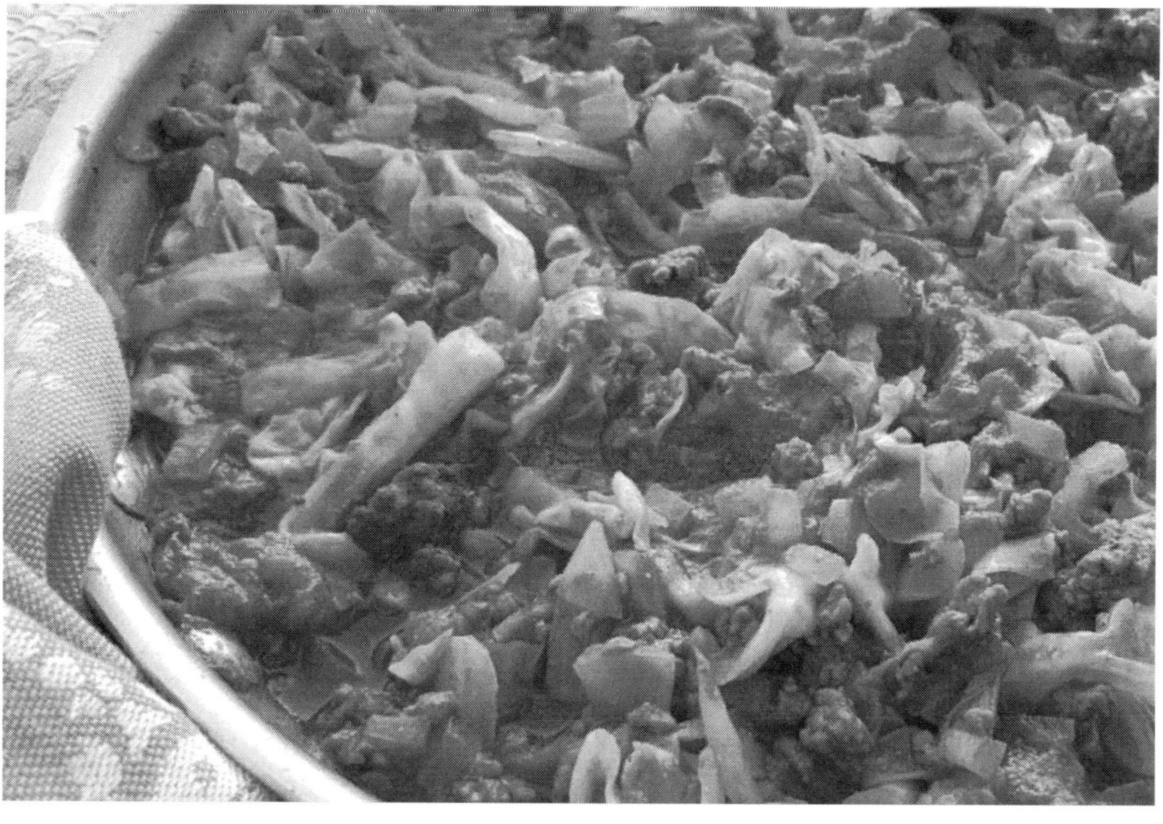

SPICY GARLIC BUTTER SHRIMP

 Cooking Difficulty: 4/10	 Cooking Time: 35 minutes	 Servings: 4

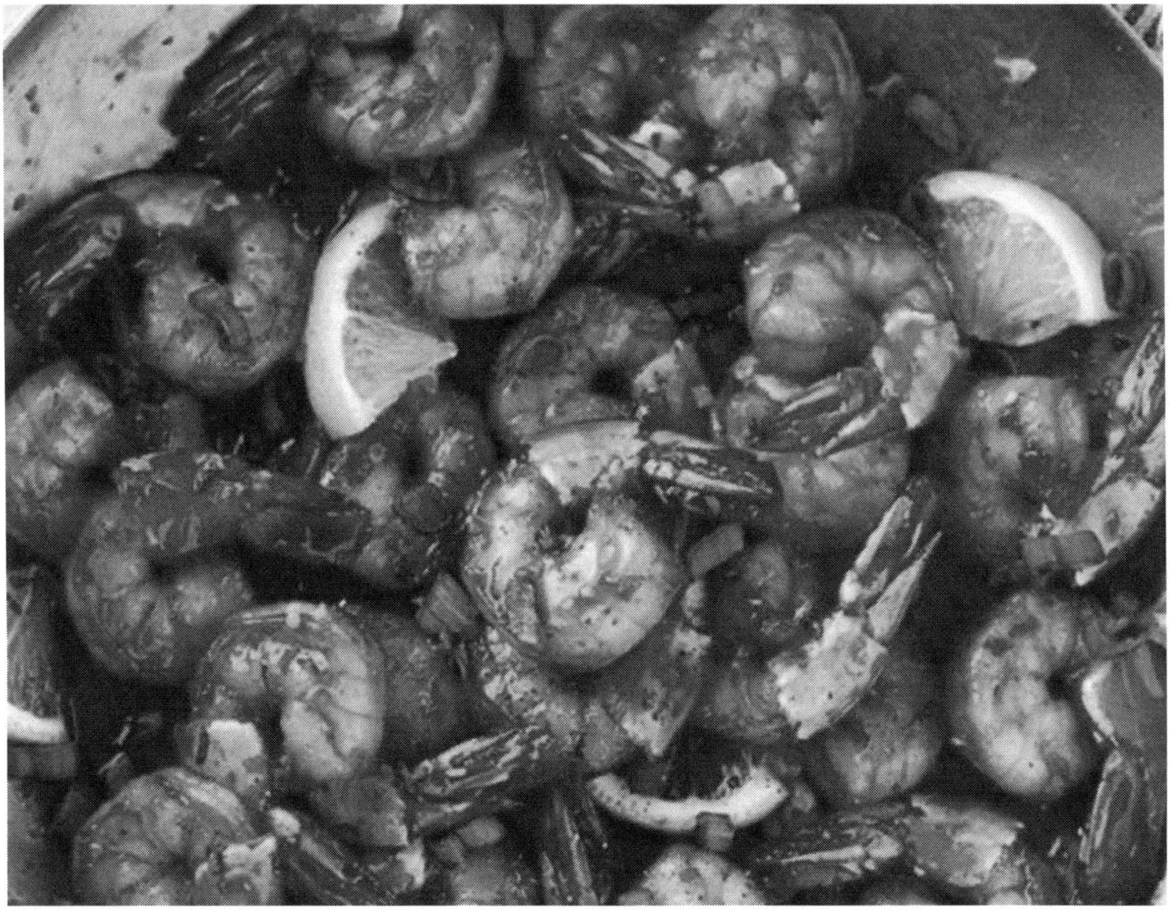

![Spicy garlic butter shrimp with lemon wedges]

NUTRITIONAL INFORMATION

300 Calories, 11g Fats, 3g Carbs, 2g Protein

INGREDIENTS

- lbs. large-sized shrimp, unpeeled
- 2 tbsps. garlic, minced
- olive oil
- lemon pepper seasoning
- garlic powder

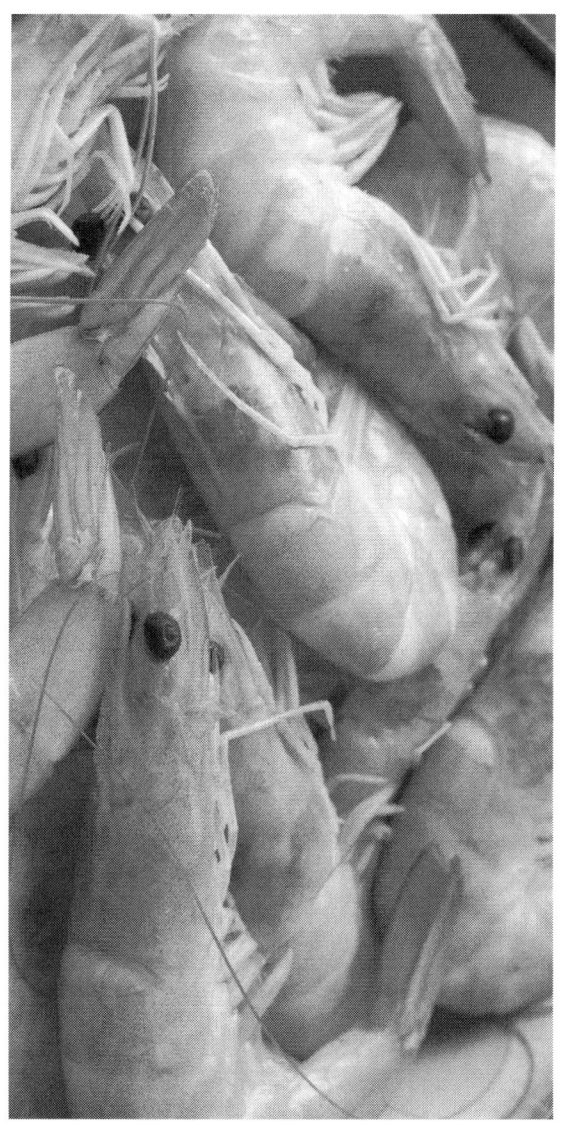

DESCRIPTION

STEP 1
Preheat the oven to 300 degrees F.

STEP 2
Mix the olive oil and the garlic.

STEP 3
Place the shrimp in a saucepan and dot with the garlic oil; sprinkle well with the garlic powder and the lemon pepper.

STEP 4
In an open state, bake for about 30 minutes, stirring once or twice, until the shrimp are opaque, making sure the shrimp is evenly cooked.

STEP 5
Serve alongside the butter sauce that is in a separate bowl or the one containing the shrimp for dipping.

STEP 6
You may serve alongside cauliflower rice. Place remaining portions in an airtight container and refrigerate for up to 2 days.

CHICKEN WITH PUMPKIN

 Cooking Difficulty: 3/10

 Cooking Time: 32 minutes

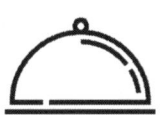 Servings: 4

INGREDIENTS

- 4 boneless chicken breasts
- 1 lb. cherry tomatoes
- 1 lb. pumpkin
- 4 crushed garlic cloves
- 2 tbsps. lemon juice
- ½ tsp. ground cumin
- ½ tsp. ground turmeric
- ½ tsp. paprika
- 2 tbsps. avocado oil
- 1 c. fresh coriander leaves

DESCRIPTION

STEP 1

Set your oven to 350 F. put the pumpkin in an ovenproof dish accompanied with the tomatoes. Sprinkle the olive oil over the vegetables and season well with salt and pepper.

STEP 2

Put the garlic, coriander, olive oil, lemon juice and spices into a food processor and blend well to make a smooth and consistent paste, then season. Coat the chicken pieces with the paste on all sides. Add chicken breasts on top of the prepared pumpkin and tomatoes. Cook for 30 minutes until meat is tender and skins are golden brown.

NUTRITIONAL INFORMATION

296.4 Calories, 5.2g Fats, 16.0g Carbs, 18.8g Protein

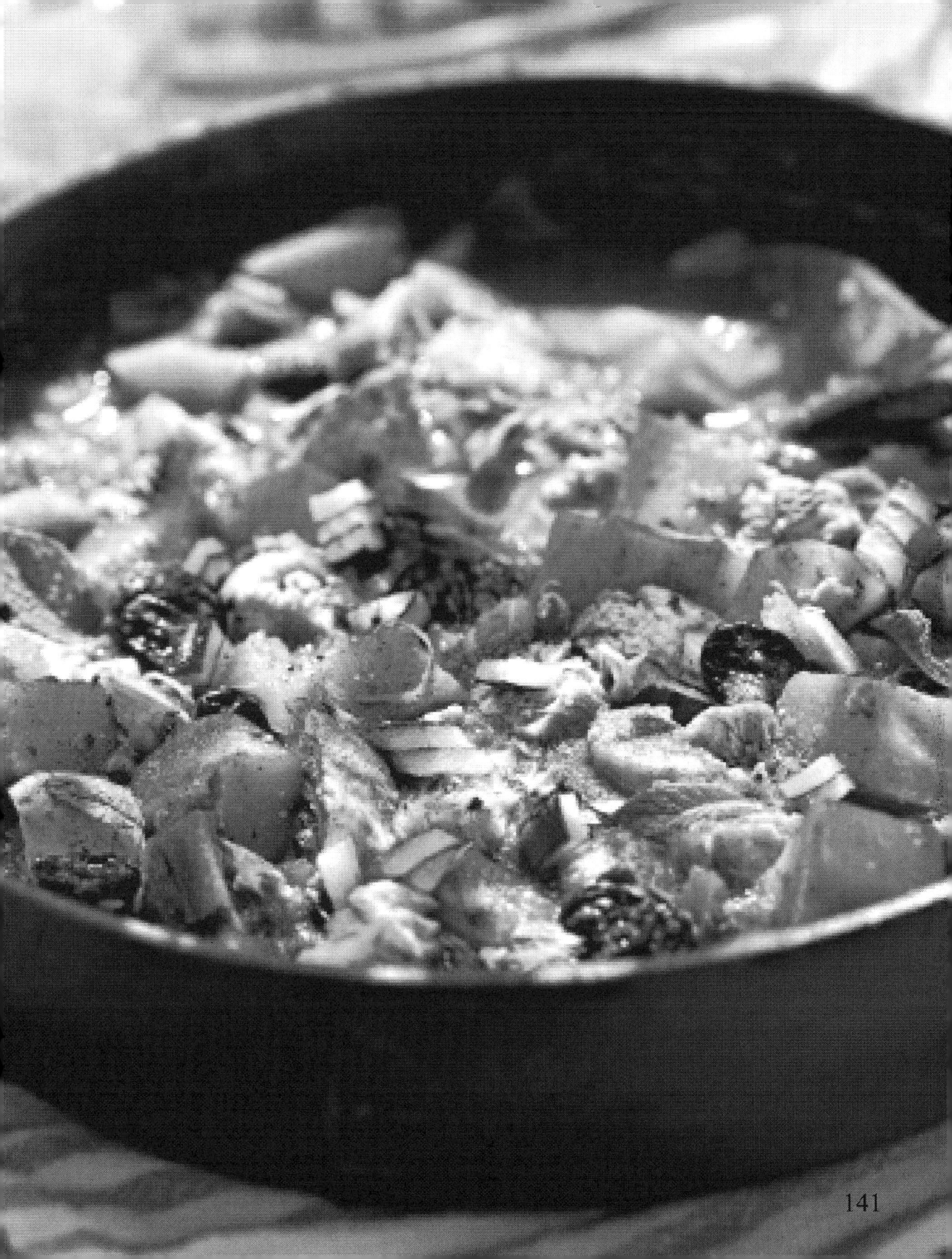

CHICKEN AND VEGGIES TORTILLA SOUP

 Cooking Difficulty: 4/10	 Cooking Time: 132 minutes	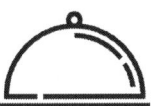 Servings: 8

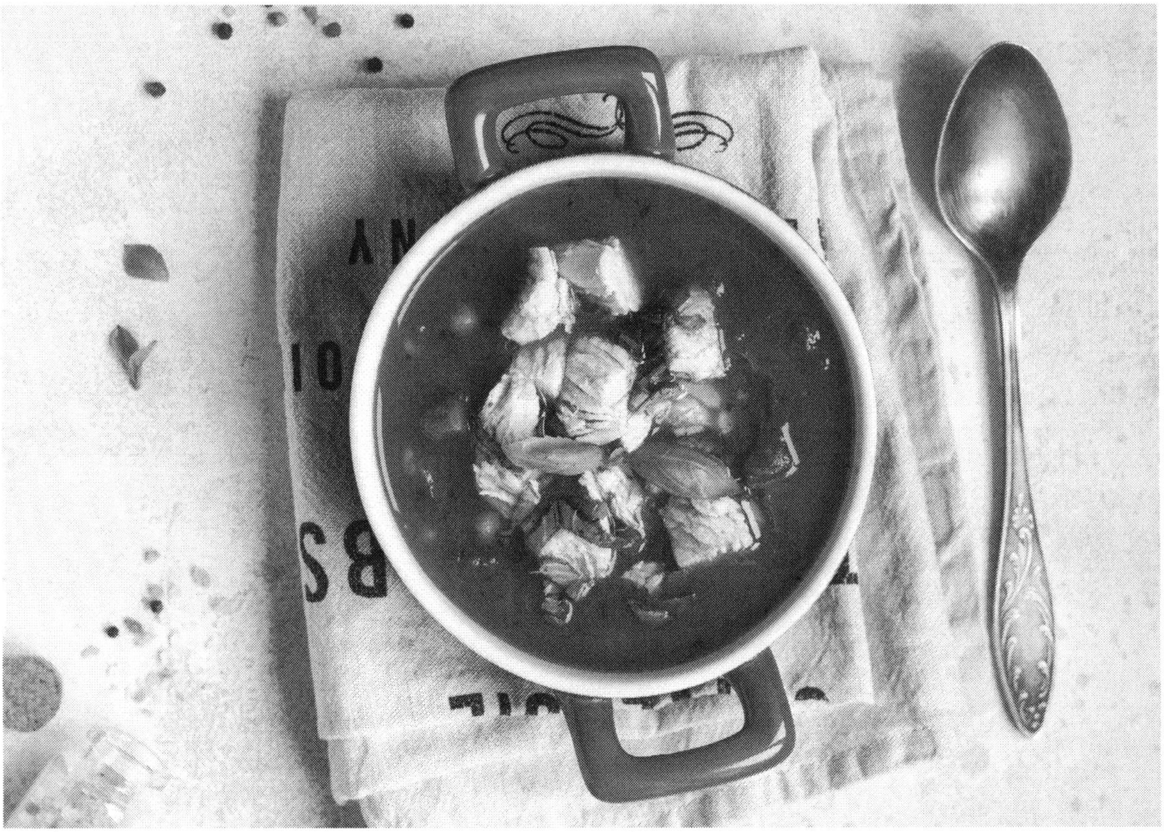

NUTRITIONAL INFORMATION

230 Calories, 8.3g Carbs, 31.6g Protein, 7.5g Fat

INGREDIENTS

- 28 oz. diced tomatoes
- 1 bunch chopped cilantro
- 1 diced sweet onion
- 1 tsp. chili powder
- 2 c. water
- 2 c. chopped celery
- 2 c. shredded carrots
- 2 chicken breasts
- 2 tbsps. tomato paste
- 32 oz. chicken broth
- 4 cloves minced garlic
- olive oil
- salt
- pepper

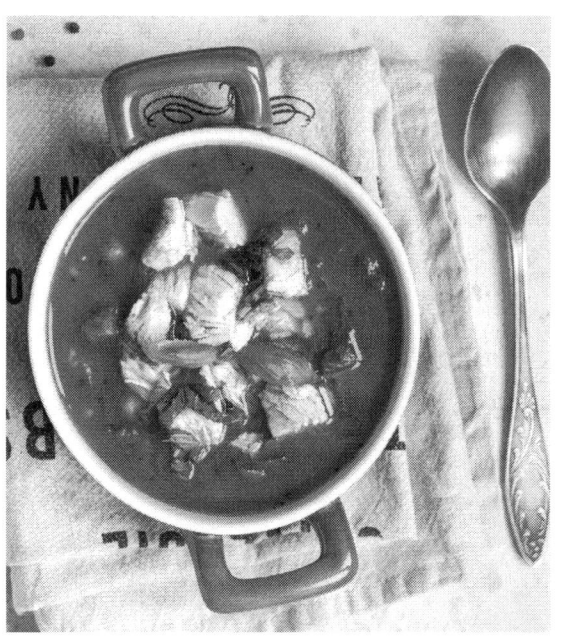

DESCRIPTION

STEP 1

Heat a large Dutch oven or crockpot over medium-high heat, add a dash of olive oil and ¼ c. of chicken broth.

STEP 2

Add garlic, salt, pepper and onion and cook until soft, adding broth as needed.

STEP 3

Add all the remaining ingredients and water to fill the pot. Cover and cook for 2 hours on low and add pepper and salt to taste if needed.

STEP 4

Shred the cooked chicken using the back of a wooden spoon and pressing it at the side of the pot. You can also use tongs or fork to break the chicken apart and shreds it.

STEP 5

Top with fresh cilantro and avocado slices. Serve.

CASHEW TURKEY MEDLEY

 Cooking Difficulty: 3/10

 Cooking Time: 23 minutes

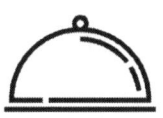 Servings: 4

INGREDIENTS

- 1 tbsp. cilantro, chopped
- black pepper
- 1 c. cashews, chopped
- 2 ½ tbsps. cashew butter
- ½ tbsp. olive oil
- ¼ c. chicken stock
- 1 onion, chopped
- 1 lb. turkey breast, skinless, deboned and cubed
- ½ tsp. sweet paprika

DESCRIPTION

STEP 1
Heat up a pan with the oil over medium-high heat, add the onion, stir and sauté for 5 minutes.

STEP 2
Add the meat and brown it for 5 minutes more.

STEP 3
Add the rest of the ingredients, toss, bring to a simmer and cook over medium heat for 30 minutes. Divide the whole mix between plates and serve.

NUTRITIONAL INFORMATION

Calories 352, Fat 12.7g, Carbs 33.2g, Protein 13.5g

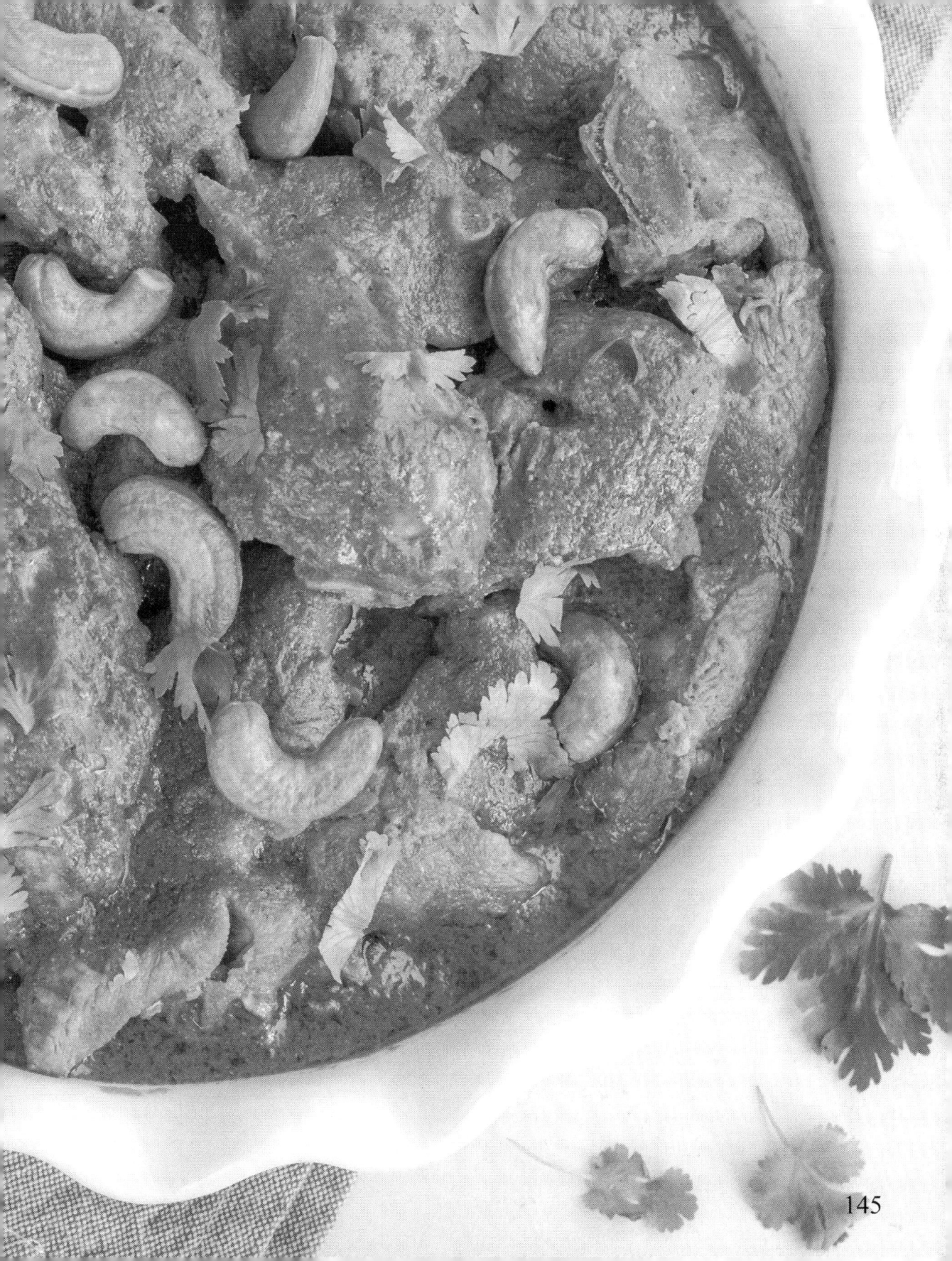

TURKEY MEATBALLS WITH TOMATO SAUCE

 Cooking Difficulty: 3/10	 Cooking Time: 25 minutes	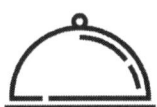 Servings: 4

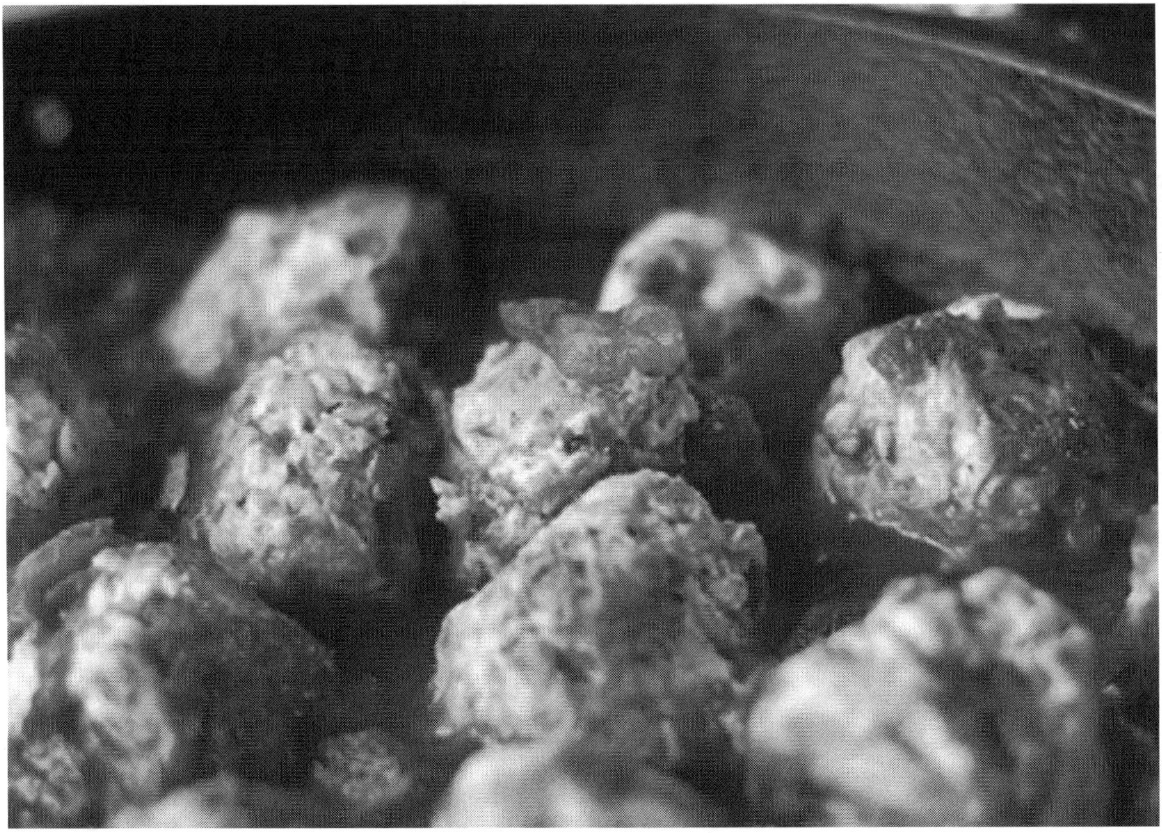

NUTRITIONAL INFORMATION

380 Calories, 26g Fats, 5g Carbs, 8g Protein

INGREDIENTS

- 7 oz. chopped fresh mushrooms
- 1 chopped onion
- 1 lightly beaten egg
- 1 tbsp. italian seasoning
- 14.5 oz. diced tomatoes
- 2 lb. lean ground turkey
- 2 tbsps. olive oil

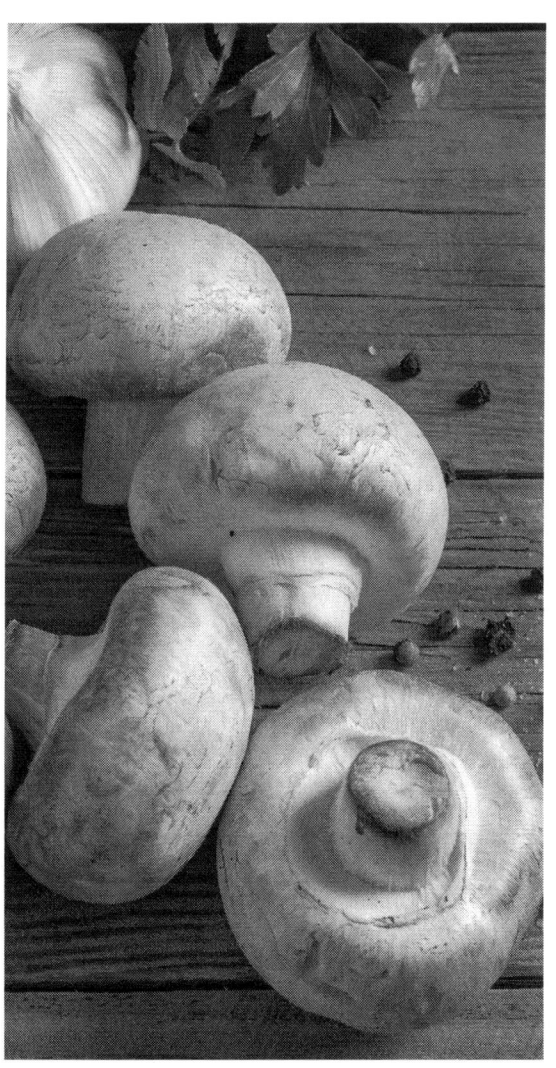

DESCRIPTION

STEP 1

In a medium-size bowl, combine mushrooms, egg, ground turkey, onion and Italian seasoning. Shape the mixture into meatballs.

STEP 2

Heat a nonstick skillet over medium heat. Add oil. Cook meatballs until brown, and there is no pink in the center or for four minutes with frequent stirring.

STEP 3

Remove from the pan and keep warm. Add tomatoes into the pan, let it boil, and simmer for 15 mins. or until thickens.

STEP 4

Add the cooked meatballs into the pan with tomatoes and simmer for around 5 minutes or until heated through.

SNACKS & DESSERTS

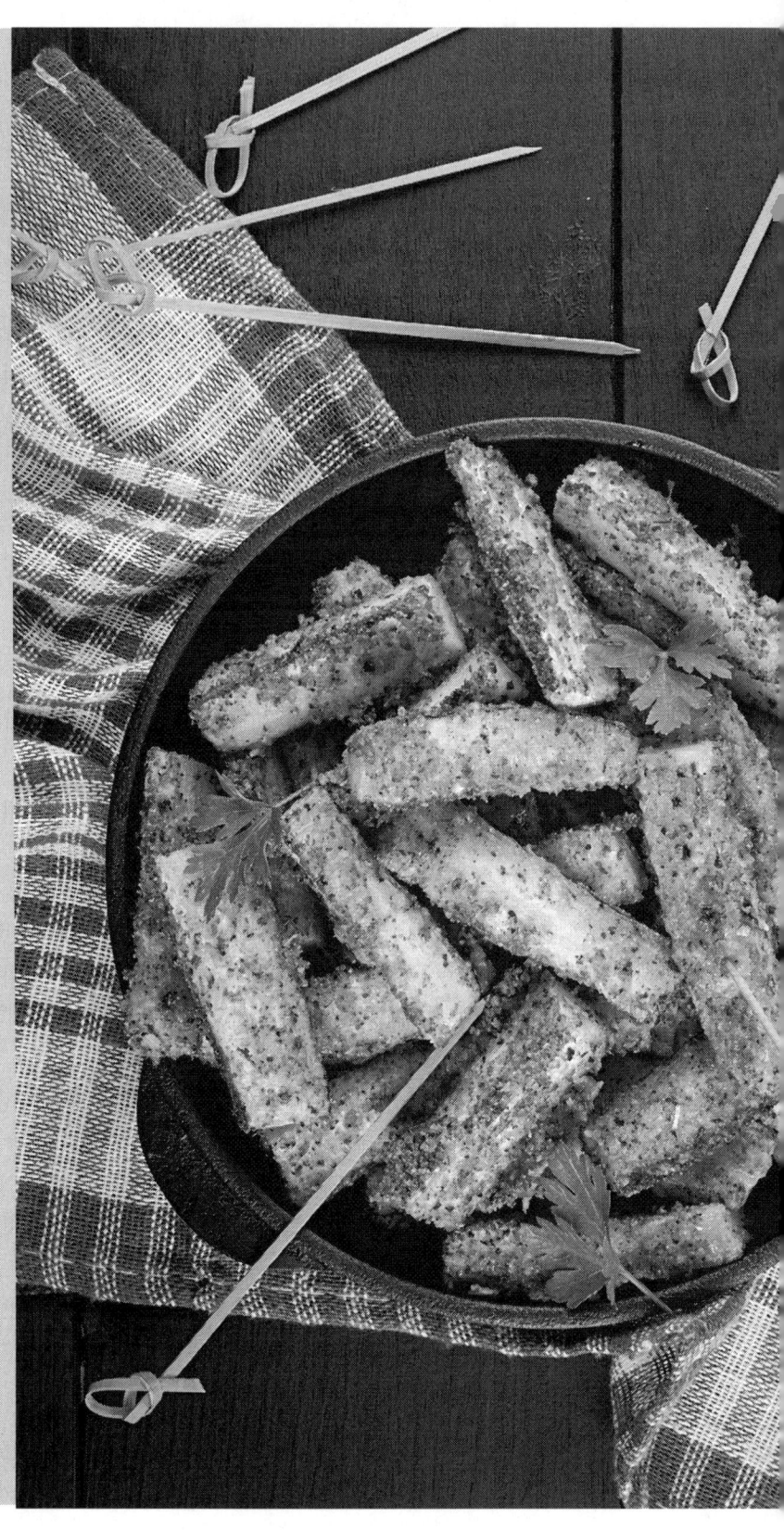

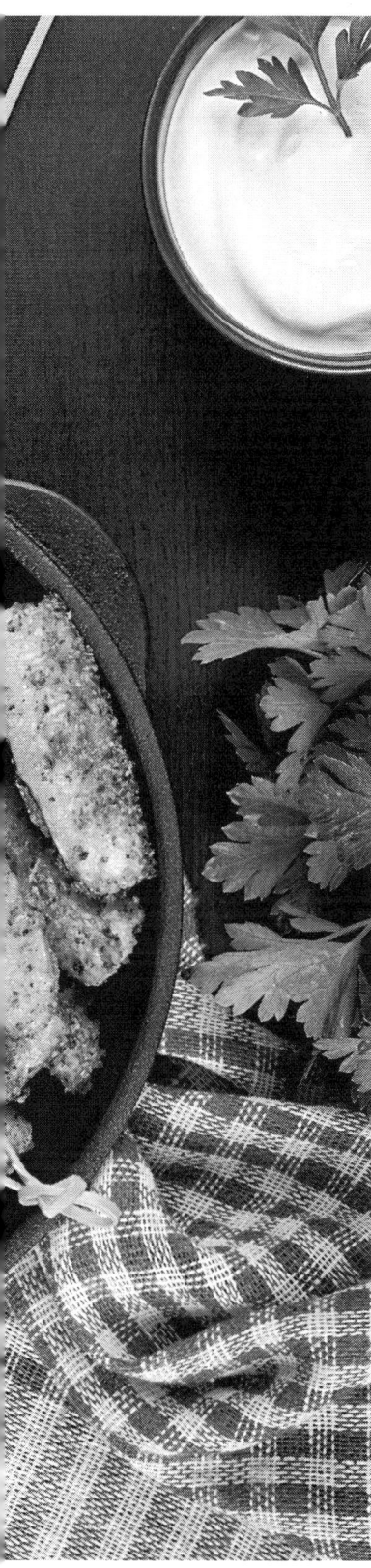

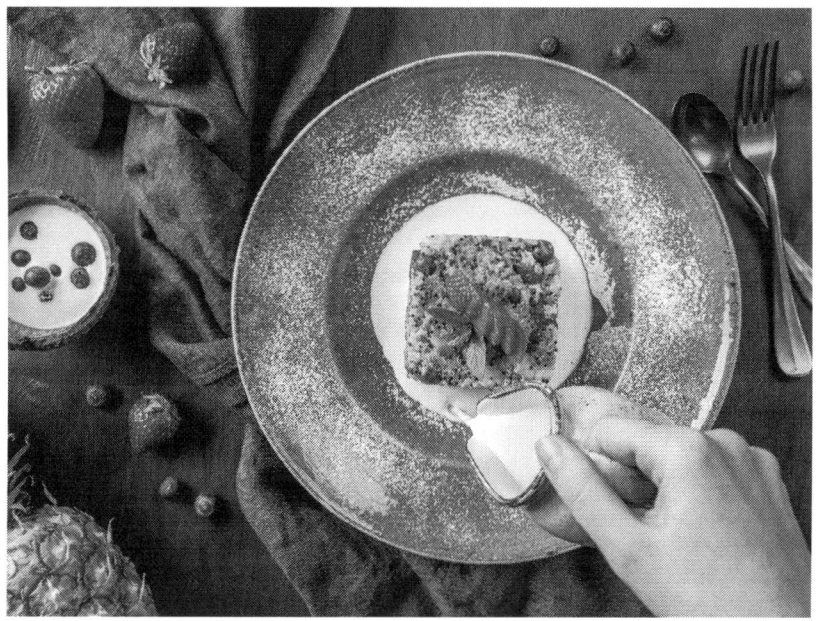

Recipes include foods recommended in the GOLO diet, such as lean sources of protein, lean dairy products, low glycemic index vegetables, whole grains, and healthy sources of fat. Recipes include low to medium GI ingredients to help maintain stable blood sugar levels.

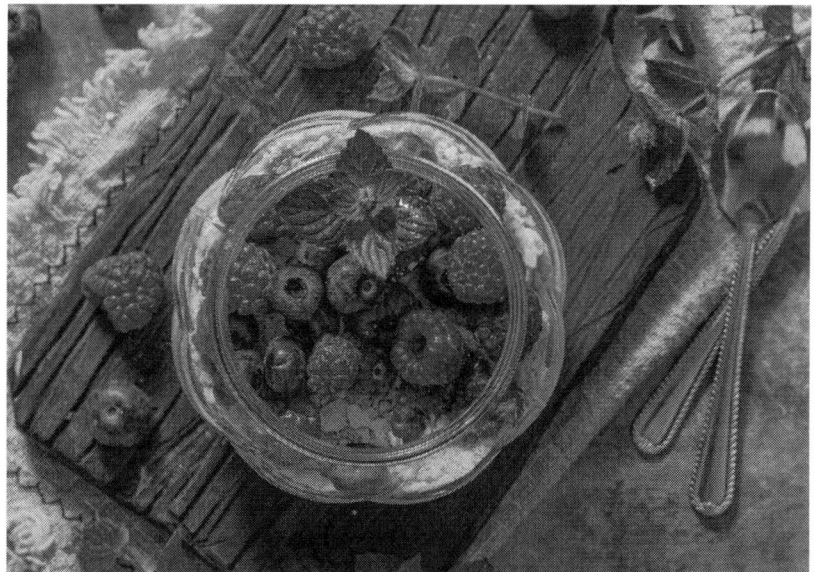

ZUCCHINI DIP

 Cooking Difficulty: 2/10

 Cooking Time: 12 minutes

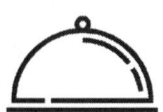 Servings: 4

INGREDIENTS

- 2 spring onions, chopped
- ¼ c. veggie stock
- 2 garlic cloves, minced
- 2 zucchinis, chopped
- 1 tbsp. olive oil
- ½ c. yogurt
- 1 tbsp. dill, chopped

DESCRIPTION

STEP 1
Heat up a pan with the oil over medium heat, add the onions and garlic, stir and sauté for 3 minutes.

STEP 2
Add the zucchinis and the other ingredients except the yogurt, toss, cook for 7 minutes more and take off the heat.

STEP 3
Add the yogurt, blend using an immersion blender, divide into bowls, and serve.

NUTRITIONAL INFORMATION

Calories 76, Fat 4.1, Carbs 7.2, Protein 3.4

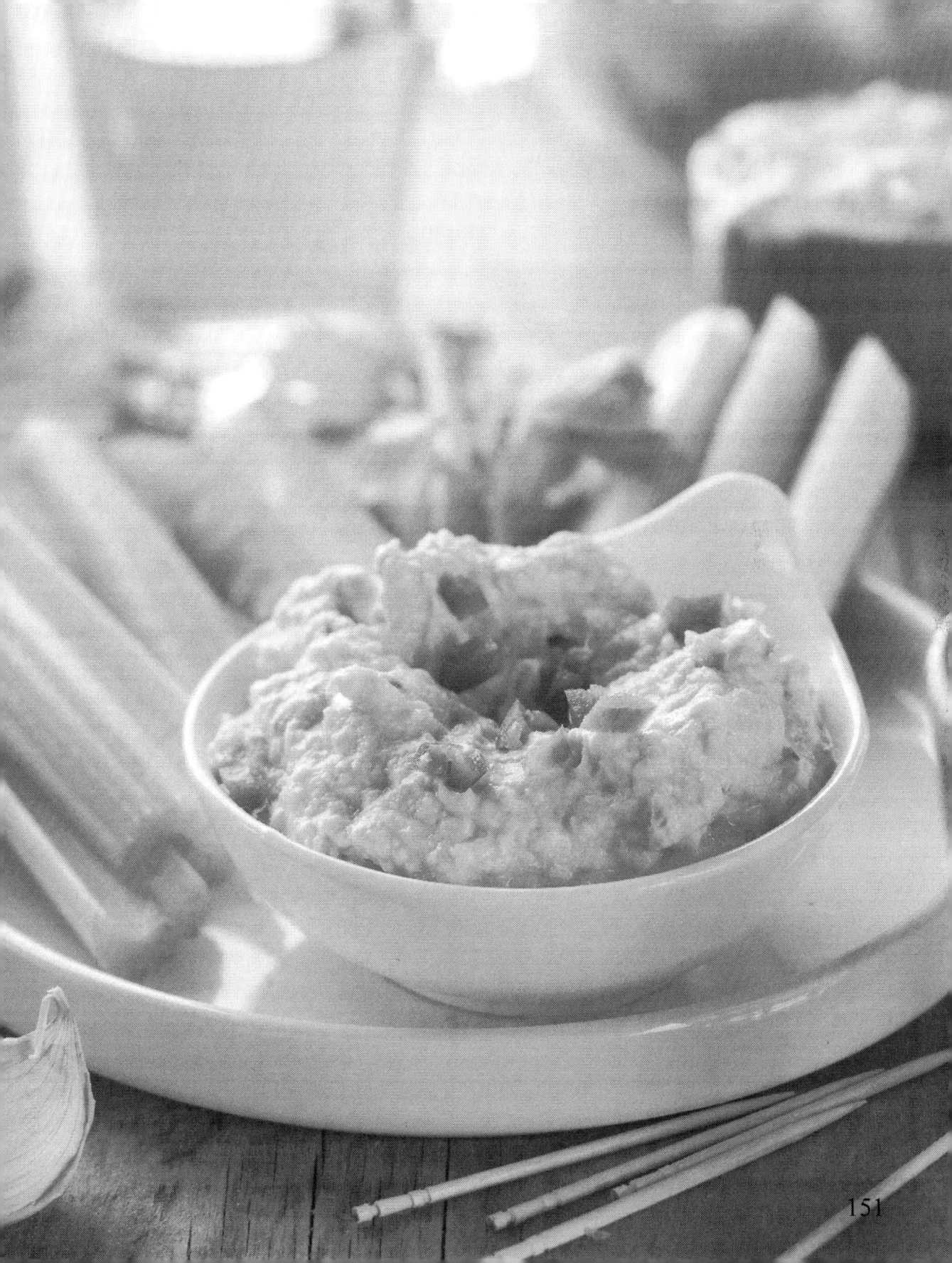

DELICIOUS HUMMUS

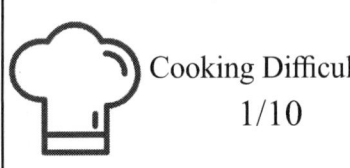 Cooking Difficulty:
1/10

 Cooking Time:
4 minutes

 Servings:
6

INGREDIENTS

- ¾ dried chickpeas
- 2 tbsps. olive oil
- 2/3 c. tahini paste
- juice of 2 lemons
- salt
- black pepper
- extra virgin olive oil for

  sprinkling

DESCRIPTION

STEP 1
Put the chickpeas in a large bowl with cold water and allow it to soak.

STEP 2
Drain and put in a saucepan with enough water to cover. Bring to a boil. Simmer on reduced heat for 1 hour, until chickpeas are soft and tender.

STEP 3
Transfer the chick-peas to a food processor and blend well to see a puree. Add in the olive oil, lemon juice, tahini paste. Mix well until smooth and consistent. Season with pepper and salt.

NUTRITIONAL INFORMATION

408 Calories, 23.6g Fats, 35.2g Net Carbs, 19.4g Protein

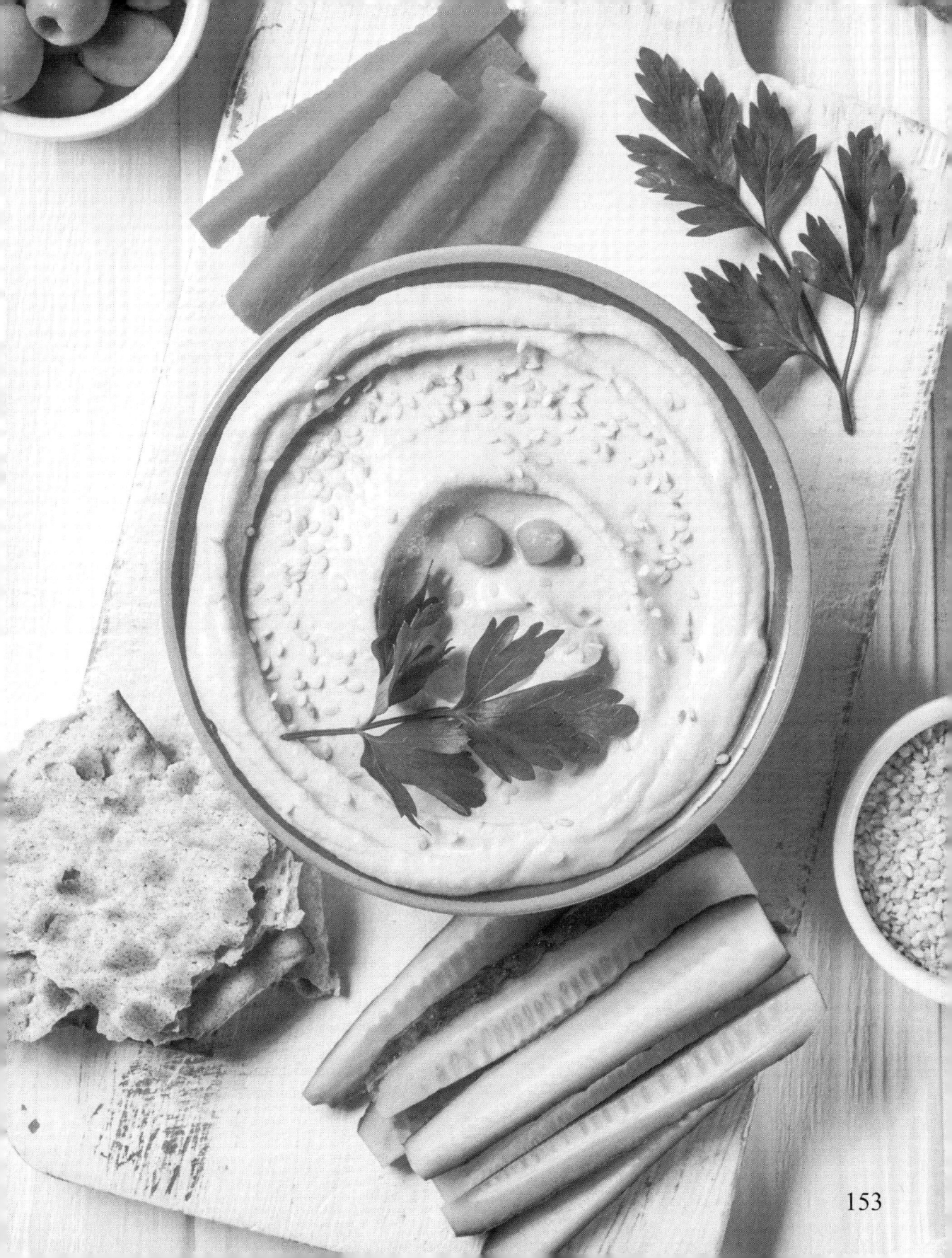

153

CAULIFLOWER POPCORN

 Cooking Difficulty: 1/10	 Cooking Time: 480 minutes	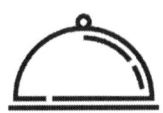 Servings: 4

INGREDIENTS

- 2 tbsps. olive oil
- 2 tsps. chili powder
- 1 tbsp. nutritional yeast
- 1 head cauliflower
- salt

DESCRIPTION

STEP 1

Before you begin making this recipe, you will want to take a few moments to cut your cauliflower into bite-sized pieces, like popcorn.

STEP 2

Once your cauliflower is set, place it into a mixing bowl and coat with the olive oil. Once coated properly, add in the nutritional yeast, salt, and the rest of the spices.

STEP 3

You can enjoy your snack immediately or place into a dehydrator at 115 for 8 hours. By doing this, it will make the cauliflower crispy! You can really enjoy it either way.

NUTRITIONAL INFORMATION

Calories: 100, Carbs: 10g, Fats: 5g, Proteins: 5g

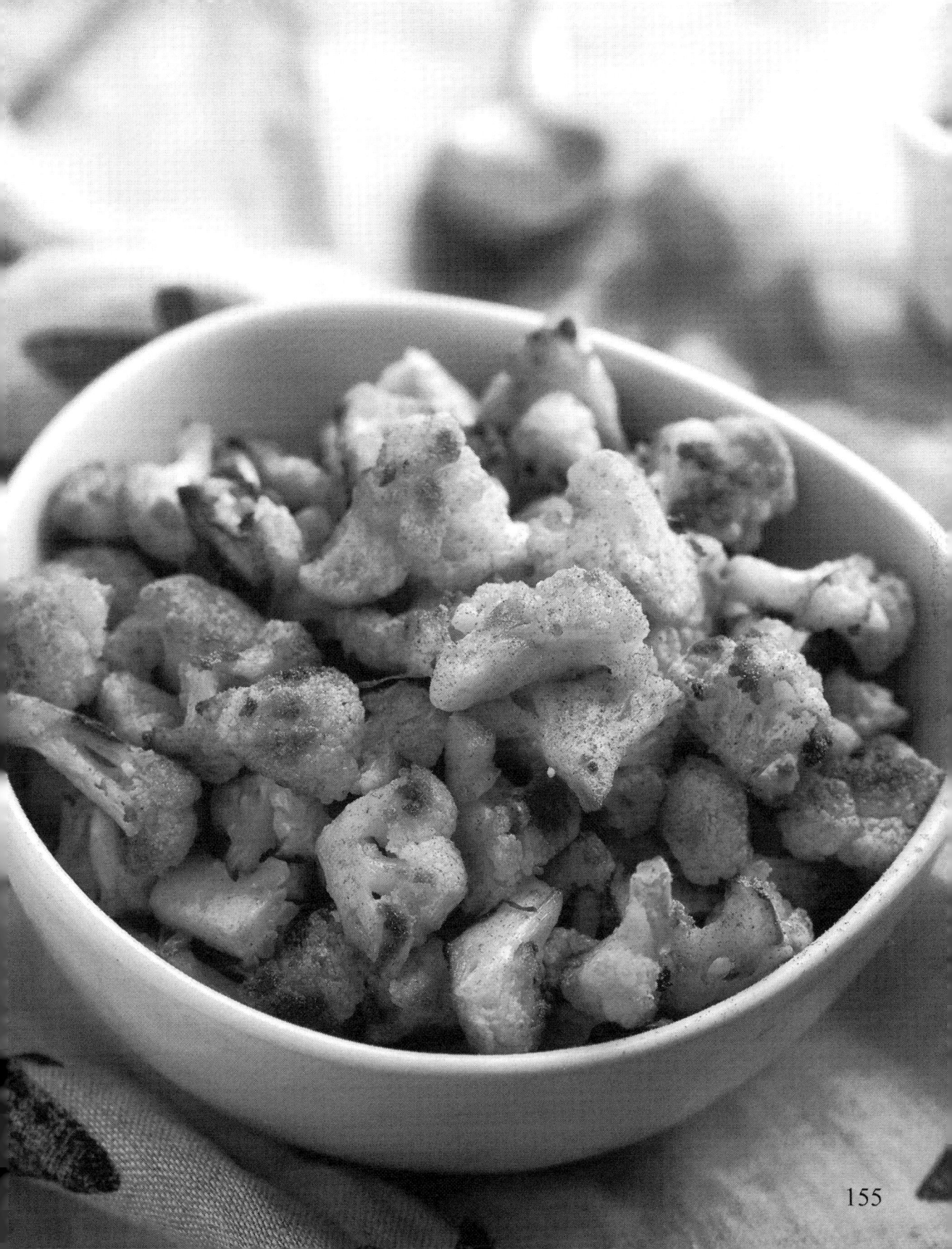

FRIED MUSHROOMS

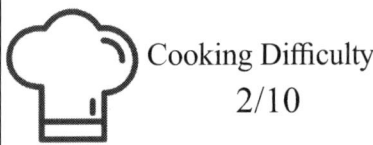 Cooking Difficulty: 2/10

 Cooking Time: 23 minutes

 Servings: 3

INGREDIENTS

- 1 lb mushrooms, halved
- 1 large onion
- 2 cloves garlic minced
- salt and pepper to taste
- 2 tablespoons of olive oil
- 1 tablespoon Worcestershire Sauce (optional)
- parsley
- italian herbs (optional)

DESCRIPTION

STEP 1
Heat a frying pan and add olive oil to it. Pour in the Worcestershire sauce.

STEP 2
Add the mushrooms and cook until golden brown, about 5 minutes. Add the onions and cook until the edges are browned and the onions are translucent. Stir in the mushrooms as they roast.

STEP 3
At the last minute, reduce the heat to low and add the crushed garlic, stirring continuously. Salt and pepper to taste. Garnish with parsley and serve.

NUTRITIONAL INFORMATION

111 Calories, 6g Fats, 3g Carbs, 6.8 Protein

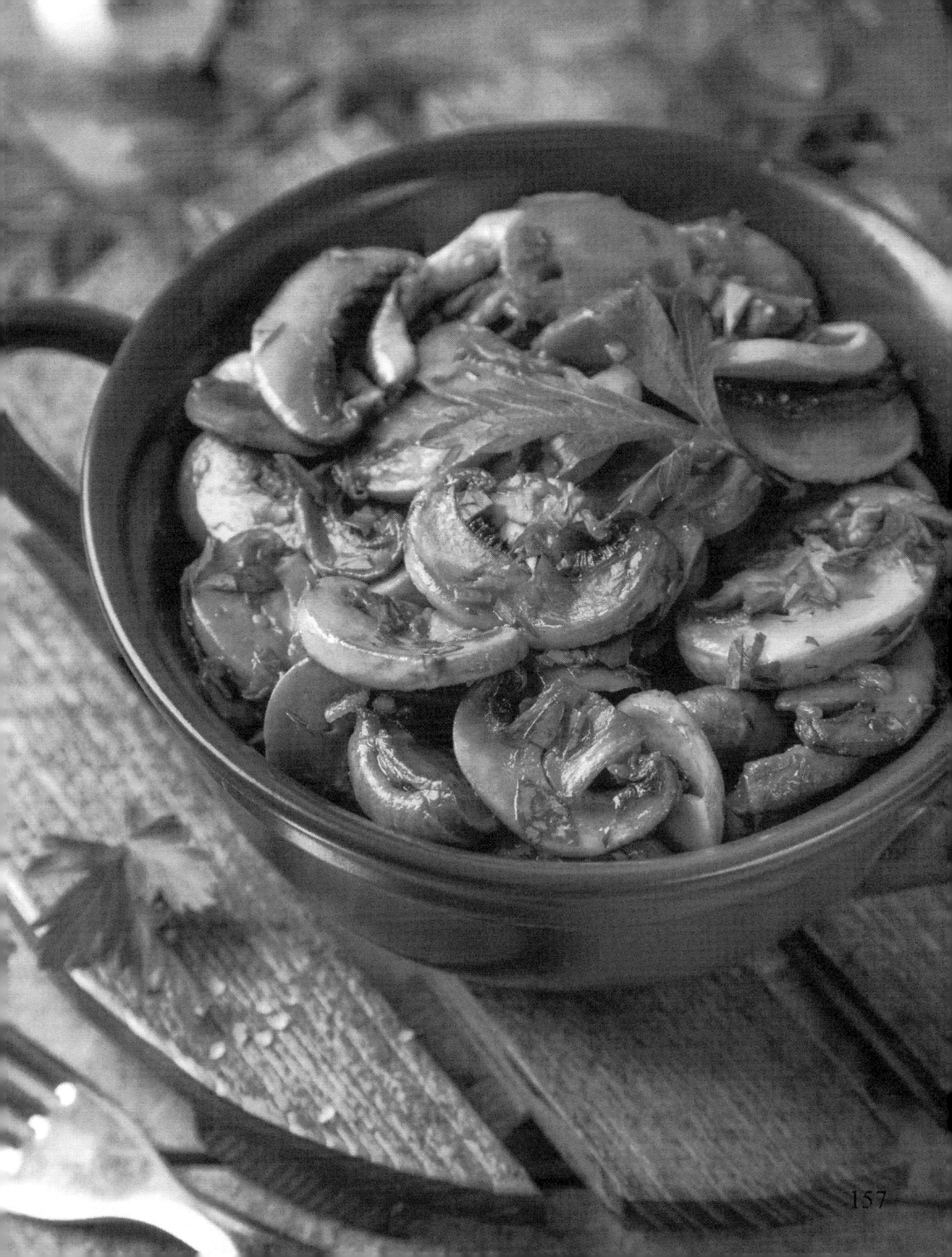

MARINATED OLIVES

 Cooking Difficulty: 1/10

 Cooking Time: 2 minutes

 Servings: 8

INGREDIENTS

- 1 1/3 c. green olives
- 4 tbsps. chopped coriander
- 1 crushed garlic clove
- 1 tsp. grated ginger
- 1 sliced red chili
- ¼ lemon

DESCRIPTION

STEP 1

Press the olives to break slightly, soak in cold water overnight, and then drain.

STEP 2

Mix well the ingredients and pour into the jars to marinade the olives. Place the jar in the fridge for at least 1 week, shaking 2-3 time.

NUTRITIONAL INFORMATION

404.7 Calories, 40.0g Fats, 13.1g Carbs, 0.5g Protein

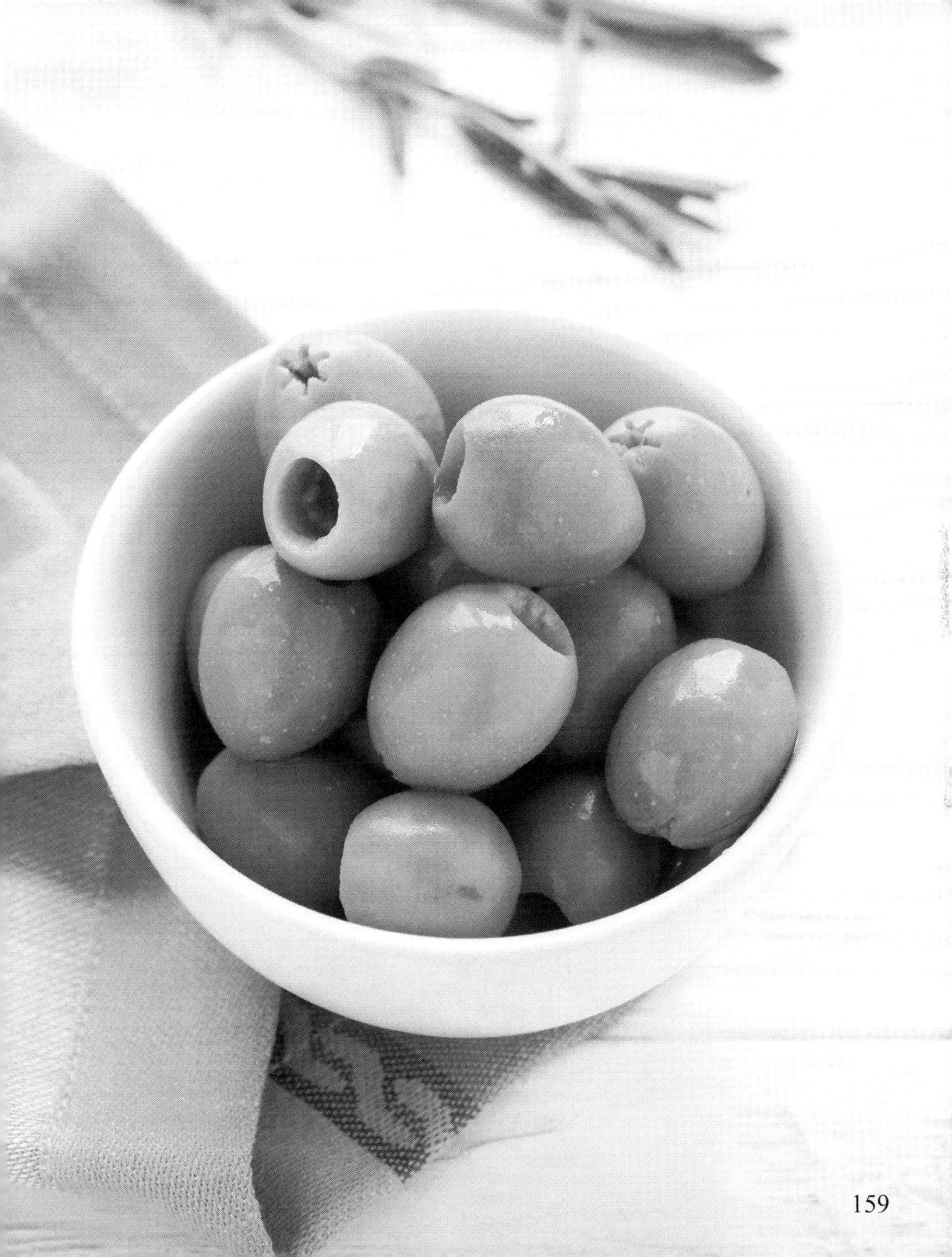

STRAWBERRY & BLUEBERRY SMOOTHIE

 Cooking Difficulty: 1/10

 Cooking Time: 1 minutes

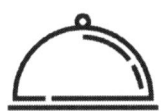 Servings: 1

INGREDIENTS

- 1/2 cup frozen strawberries
- 1 cup blueberries
- blackberry optional
- 6 ice cubes

DESCRIPTION

STEP 1
Using a blender, set in all your ingredients and blend until very smooth. Enjoy.

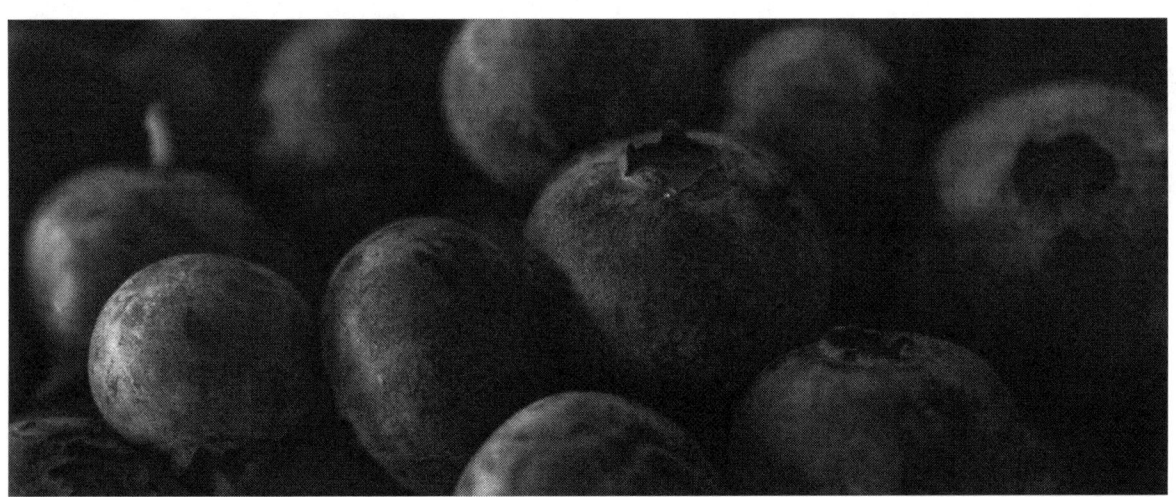

NUTRITIONAL INFORMATION

Calories: 330, Carbs: 6 g, Fat: 8.8 g, Protein: 6.9 g

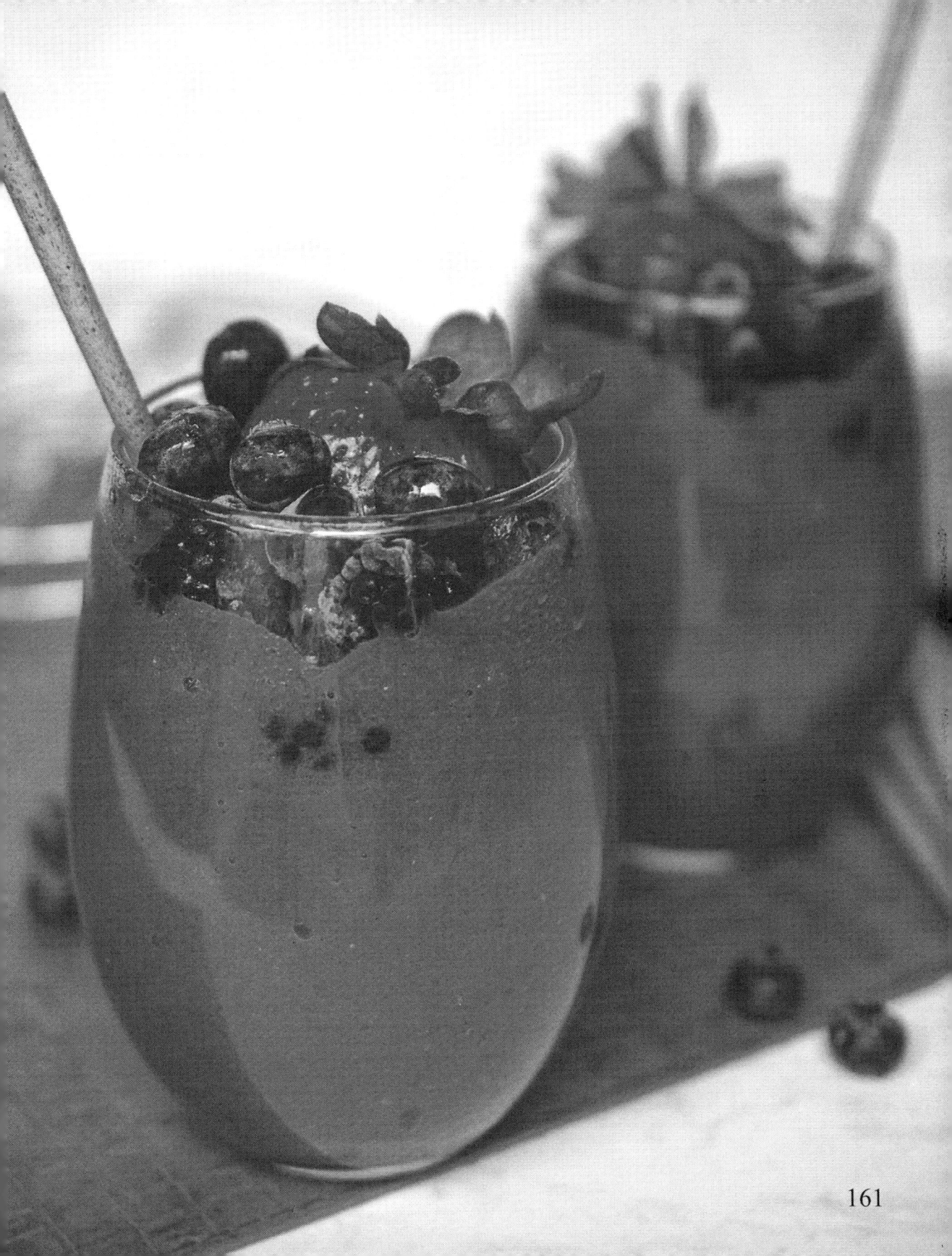

RAINBOW FRUIT SALAD

 Cooking Difficulty: 1/10	 Cooking Time: 5 minutes	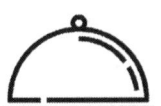 Servings: 4

INGREDIENTS

for the fruit salad:
- 1 lb. hulled strawberries, sliced
- 1 c. kiwis, halved, cubed
- 1 ¼ c. blueberries
- 1 1/3 c. blackberries
- 1 c. pineapple chunks

for the maple lime dressing:
- 2 tsps. lime zest
- 1 tbsp. lime juice

DESCRIPTION

STEP 1
Prepare the salad, and for this, take a bowl, place all its ingredients and toss until mixed.

STEP 2
Prepare the dressing, and for this, take a small bowl, place all its ingredients and whisk well.

STEP 3
Drizzle the dressing over salad, toss until coated and serve.

NUTRITIONAL INFORMATION

Calories: 88.1, Fat: 0.4 g, Carbs: 22.6 g, Protein: 1.1 g

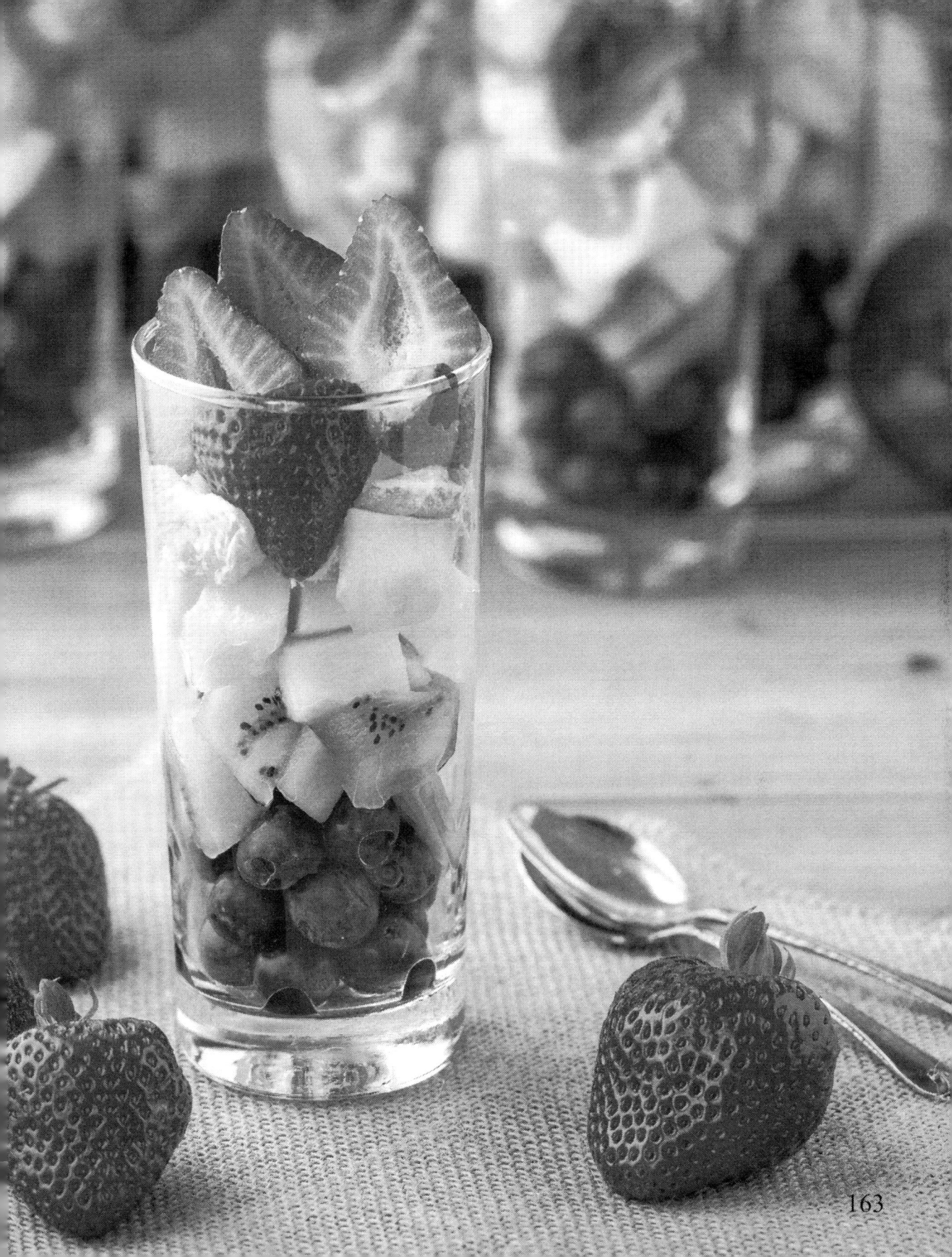

KALE DIP

 Cooking Difficulty: 2/10

 Cooking Time: 22 minutes

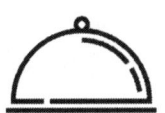 Servings: 4

INGREDIENTS

- 1 tsp. chili powder
- 1 c. coconut cream
- 1 tbsp. olive oil
- ¼ tsp. black pepper
- 1 bunch kale leaves
- 1 shallot, chopped

DESCRIPTION

STEP 1
Heat up a pan with the oil over medium heat, add the shallots, stir and sauté for 4 minutes.

STEP 2
Add the kale and the other ingredients, bring to a simmer, and cook over medium heat for 16 minutes.

STEP 3
Blend using an immersion blender, divide into bowls and serve as a snack.

NUTRITIONAL INFORMATION

Calories 188, Fat 17.9g, Carbs 7.6g, Protein 2.5g

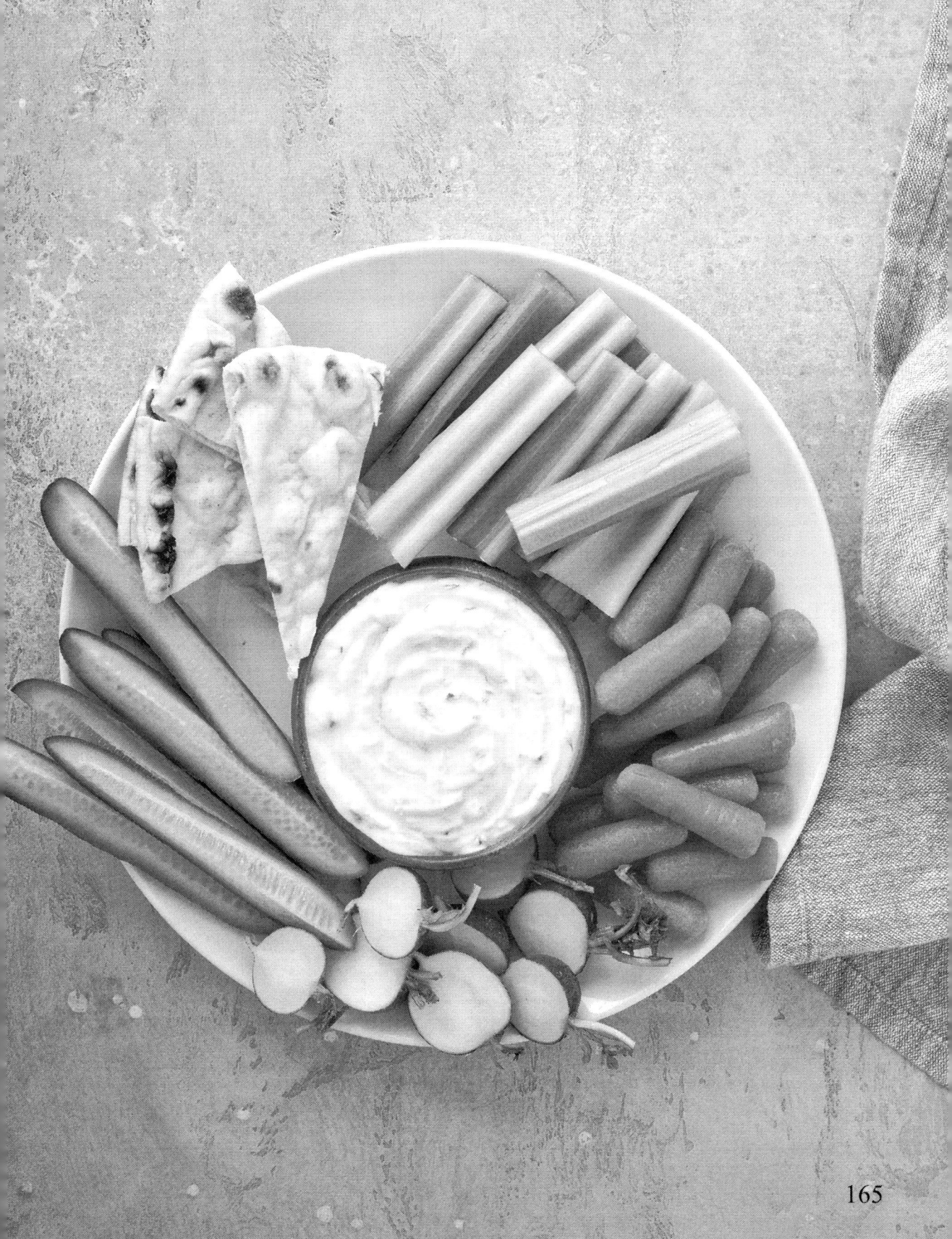

COCONUT BLACKBERRY SMOOTHIE

 Cooking Difficulty: 1/10

 Cooking Time: 1 minutes

 Servings: 1

INGREDIENTS

- 1/2 cup coconut milk
- 1/2 cup blackberries
- 2 tablespoons shredded coconut
- 5 mint leaves
- 5 cashews

DESCRIPTION

STEP 1
Using a blender, set in all your ingredients and blend until very smooth. Enjoy.

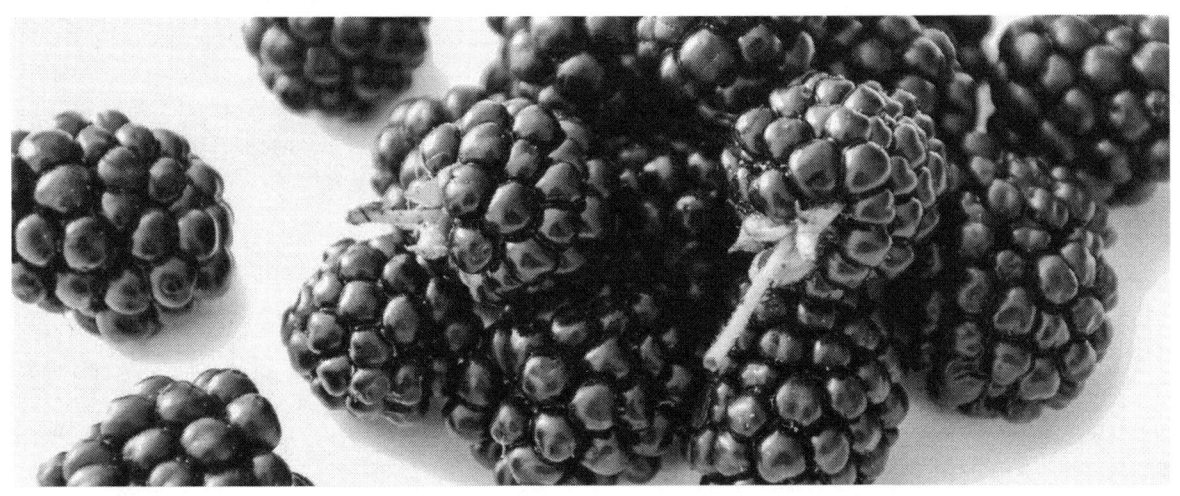

NUTRITIONAL INFORMATION

Calories: 321, Fat: 19.9 g, Carbs: 7.2 g, Protein: 7 g

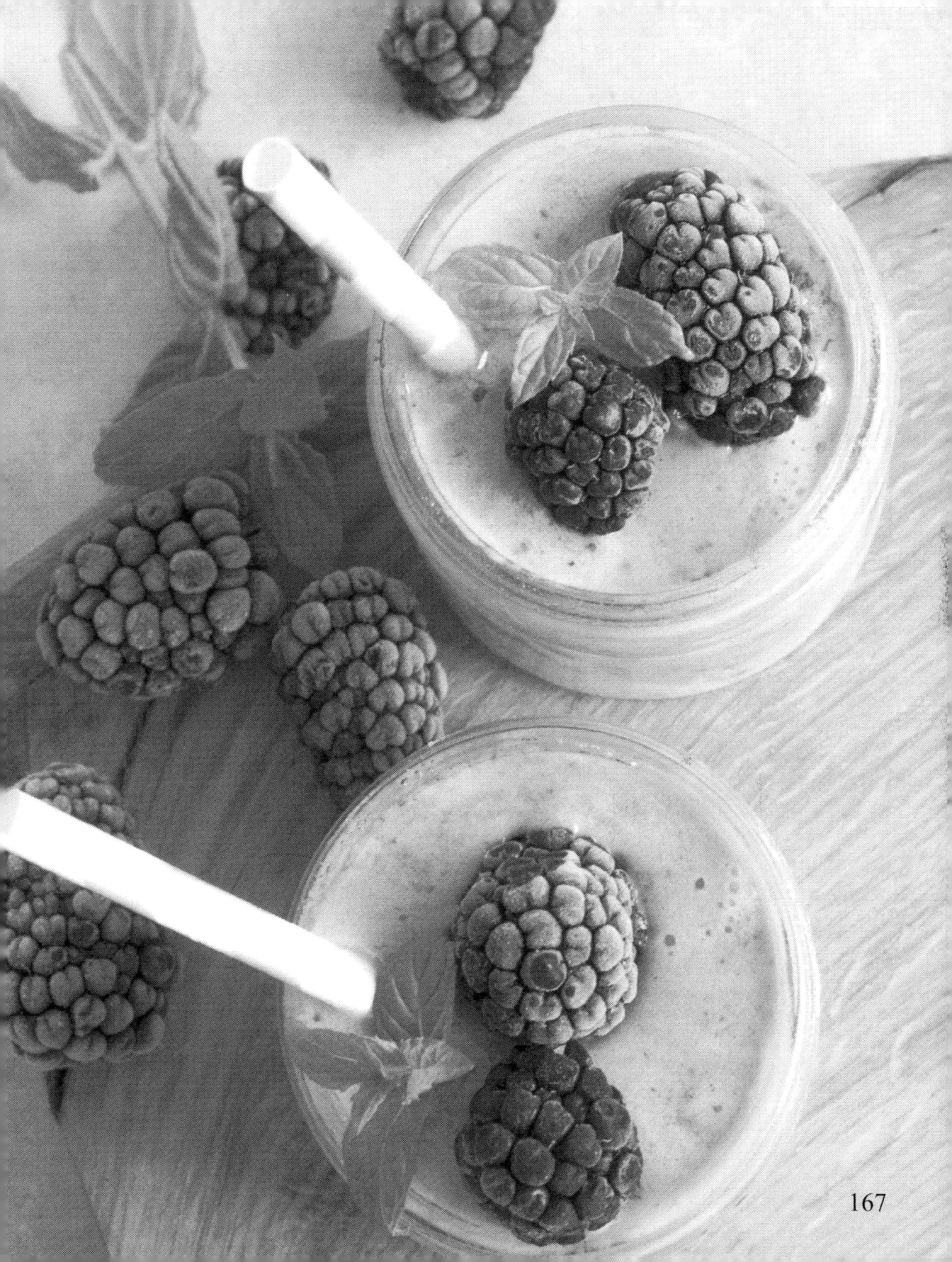

KALE AND ALMONDS

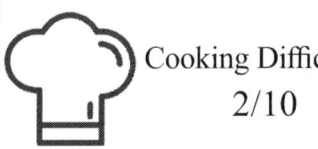 Cooking Difficulty: 2/10

 Cooking Time: 8 minutes

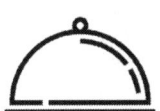 Servings: 4

INGREDIENTS

- 1 c. water
- 1 big kale bunch, chopped
- 1 tbsp. balsamic vinegar
- 1/3 c. toasted almonds
- 3 minced garlic cloves
- 1 small chopped yellow onion
- 2 tbsps. olive oil

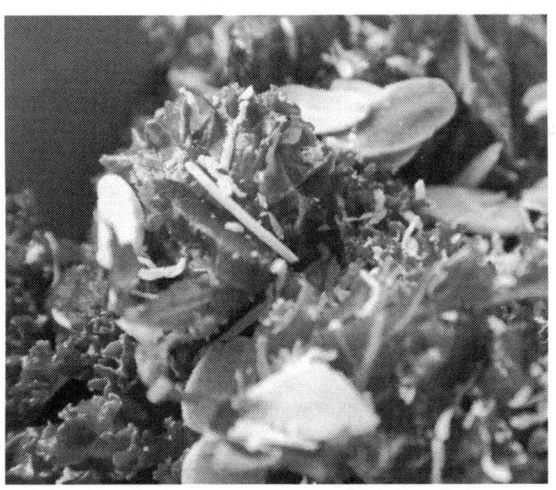

DESCRIPTION

STEP 1
Set your instant pot on sauté mode, add oil, heat it up, add onion, stir and cook for 3 minutes.

STEP 2
Add garlic, water and kale, stir, cover and cook on High for 4 minutes.

STEP 3
Add salt, pepper, vinegar, and almonds, toss well, divide between plates and serve as a side dish.

STEP 4
Enjoy!

NUTRITIONAL INFORMATION

140 Calories, 6g Fat, 1g Carbs, 3g Protein

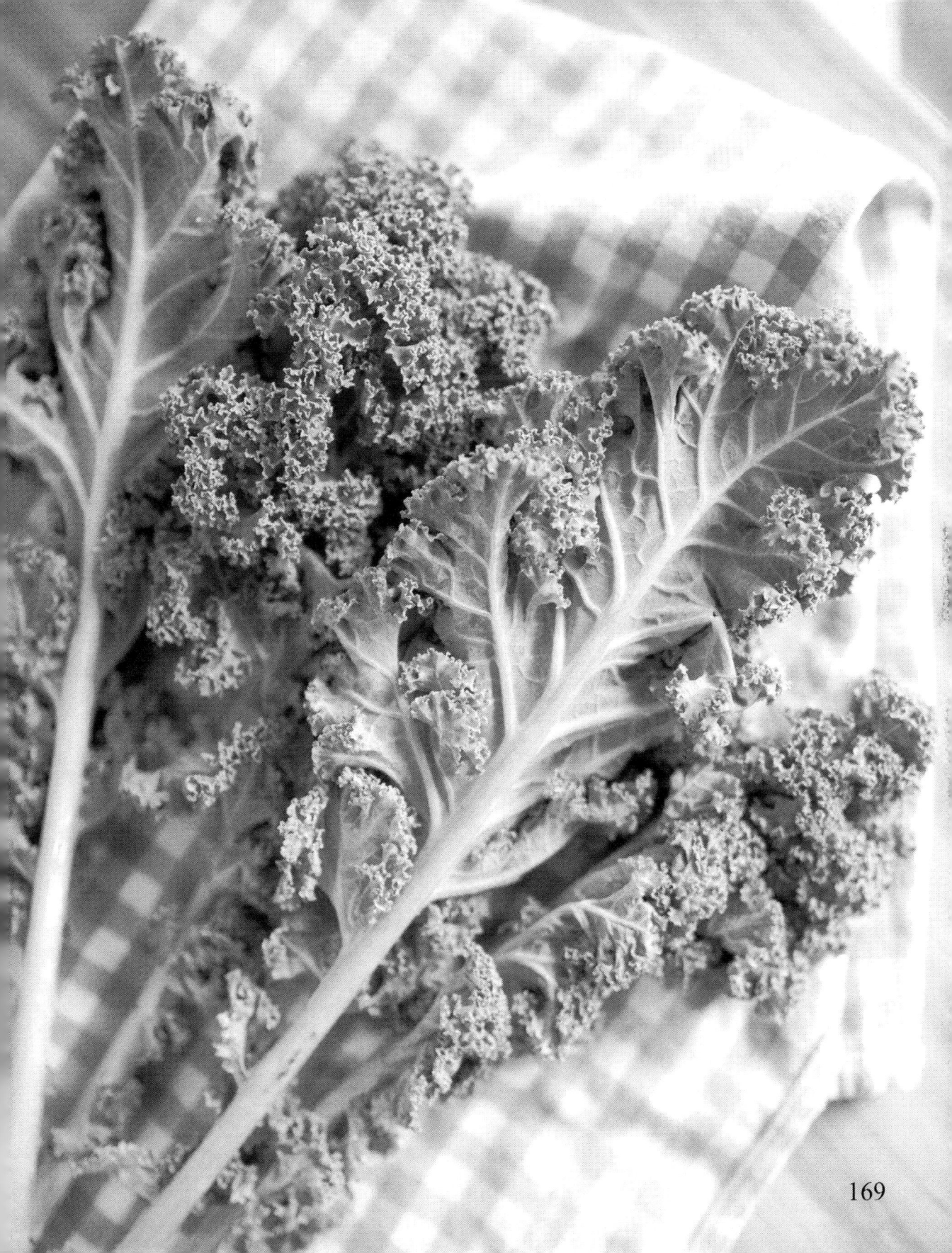

CONCLUSION

As you embark on your GOLO Diet journey, remember that it is a process of self-discovery and growth. Embrace the challenges and celebrate the victories along the way. With dedication, determination, and the knowledge gained from this book, you are equipped to make positive changes and achieve your goals.

Here's to a healthier, happier you on the path to GOLO success!

Henry Irving

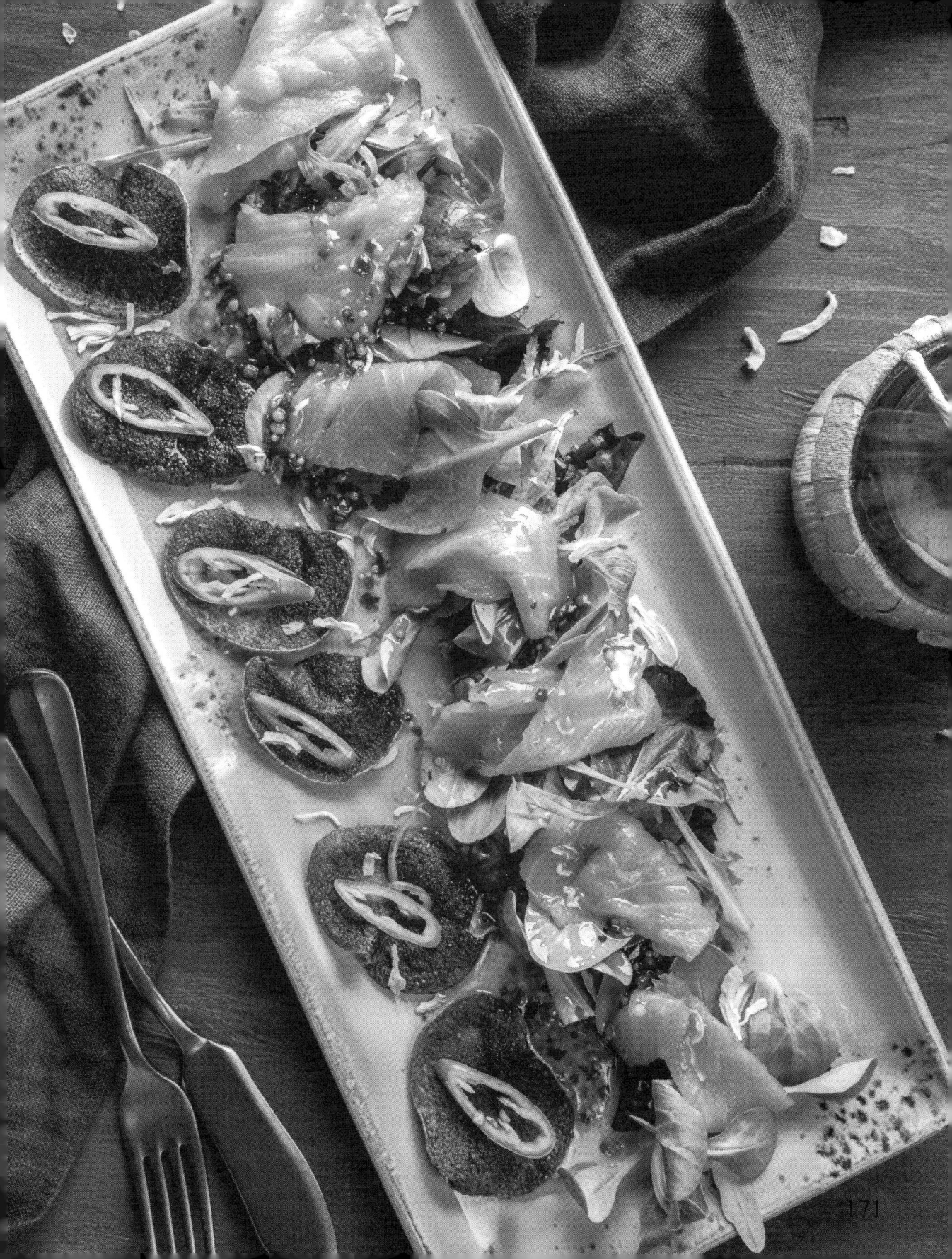

Made in United States
Troutdale, OR
09/03/2023

12587715R00095